NEONATAL MEDICINE

MALCOLM L. CHISWICK

MD, MRCP, DCH

Consultant-in-Charge of
the Special Care Baby Unit and
Regional Neonatal Intensive Care
Unit, St Mary's Hospital,
Manchester

UPDATE BOOKS

LONDON/NEW JERSEY

Published by

UPDATE PUBLICATIONS LIMITED

Available in the United Kingdom and Eire in paperback only from

Update Publications Ltd
33/34 Alfred Place
London WC1E 7DP
England

Available outside the United Kingdom in hardbound edition only from

Update Publishing International, Inc.
2337 Lemoine Avenue
Fort Lee, New Jersey 07024
USA

First published 1978

British Library Cataloguing in Publication Data

Chiswick, Malcolm L
  Neonatal medicine.
  1. Infants (Newborn) – Diseases
  I. Title
  618.9'201   RJ254

  ISBN 0–906141–01–X

ISBN 0 906141 01 X

Printed and bound in Great Britain by
Morrison & Gibb Ltd, London and Edinburgh

Contents

To Claire, Linton and Lindsey-Jane

Adaptation

*He came too soon
Into this place
And now he struggles to adapt.
No cradle for him,
Instead a shell of perspex pierced by tangled wires
To assist his survival.*

*Will he remember
When senescence comes
And once more with grunting breath he struggles to adapt
To another place?*

M.L.C.

Foreword

THERE have been many important advances in our knowledge of the physiology and pathology of the neonate in the past two decades and many of them have been from the work of British investigators. Their application to the care of new-born babies has, however, not been universal and our perinatal practice remains almost archaic in some respects. The consequence of the characteristic British failure to put theory into practice has been that the general rate of improvement in our care of new-born babies in terms of humanity, morbidity and mortality has been less than it could have been and less than has been achieved elsewhere. This has been due not so much to a lack of intensive care facilities as to a failure to adapt routine practices to our growing knowledge of a baby's emotional and physiological needs.

There are a number of excellent books on neonatology for specialists in this field, but there has been a need for an up-to-date, down-to-earth text which could be read at a sitting and which makes clear to the occasional neonatologist, whether he or she be a general practitioner, a paediatric or obstetric resident or a midwife, how common problems should be handled in the light of current knowledge.

I believe that my colleague, Dr Malcolm Chiswick, one of a growing corps of specialised neonatologists working to improve our knowledge and standards of practice in this field, has given us such a text. I have no doubt that this book could have a great influence on the way our babies are looked after—particularly at birth and on their discharge from hospital. Sensible care—not special care or intensive care—is what most babies need.

Professor J. A. Davis
Department of Child Health,
University of Manchester

Preface

ALTHOUGH mortality and morbidity during the neonatal period are greater than at any other time in childhood, medical students in many countries complete their undergraduate training in paediatrics without having received adequate teaching in neonatology. It is not surprising that the paediatric resident may feel unsure of himself when asked to manage an unwell newborn baby.

The policy of hospital confinement may deprive the family practitioner of contact with newborn babies and he may become unfamiliar with their problems. The practice of early discharge from the maternity hospital means that the family practitioner may be called upon to give primary care to a neonate he has not seen before.

The midwife and neonatal nurse are in a unique position to make an early diagnosis of disorders in the newborn because of their hour-to-hour contact with mothers and babies in the delivery unit, postnatal ward and neonatal nursery. However, nursing procedures and policies are often carried out without the nurse or midwife properly understanding the underlying physiological needs of the neonate in sickness and in health.

It is with these teaching problems in mind that I have endeavoured to write a short text on neonatal medicine that is a blend of theory and clinical practice and that recognises the continuum of fetal and neonatal life. It originally appeared as a series of articles in *Update*, and the intended audience for the articles was composed mainly of family practitioners. It became clear, however, that the articles were being read also by medical students, hospital doctors and midwives. The author and publishers received many requests for reprints of the articles, and the concept of a book containing updated versions of the articles was developed.

I am grateful to Professor J. A. Davis for his encouragement in this venture. I thank the Department of Medical Illustration, University of Manchester, Professor C. R. Whitfield and Dr J. G. B. Russell for supplying some of the illustrative material. It is a pleasure to acknowledge the help of my secretary, Mrs Louise Farrow, and of Update Publications. Finally, I wish to thank my wife and children for being tolerant and understanding when business encroached upon family activities.

Malcolm L. Chiswick
February 1978

1. Care of the Unborn Baby

THE aetiology of virtually all neonatal disease lies with events that operate before or during birth. The fetal milieu is adversely influenced by poor socioeconomic circumstances and much remains to be learned about the complex interrelation between the underprivileged mother and her disadvantaged fetus. Better living standards and improved antenatal and intrapartum care have contributed to the downward trend in stillbirth and in perinatal and neonatal mortality rates in the last 20 to 30 years (Figure 1). The fetus is becoming increasingly exposed to technology both before and during birth and in many countries there has been a sharp decline in the incidence of home deliveries. This changing pattern of obstetric management may deny the family practitioner the experience of continuity of care from conception through birth to the neonatal period.

Care of the unborn baby involves clinical management based on the results of fetal assessment. In the majority of cases clinical management will be governed by a policy of non-intervention, allowing the mother to be delivered of her baby at term by the vaginal route. There are numerous methods of fetal assessment and no single test, however sophisticated, can provide the clinician with all the information he requires. The efficacy of a particular test depends on the clinician's skill in interpreting the result. The following questions have to be answered:

1. Can the fetus safely be left *in utero* pending further assessment?

2. Should the fetus be removed from a hostile intra-uterine environment to preserve his or her life?

3. Should the fetal environment be manipulated in any way to preserve life?

4. Should the fetus be aborted (in the case of certain congenital abnormalities)?

A particular test may yield information concerning fetal size, maturity, antepartum health or intrapartum health. The interplay of these factors is shown in Figure 2. Growth is a function of size and maturity. Suboptimal fetal growth implies poor fetal health, which in turn may compromise the fetus during the stress of labour and delivery.

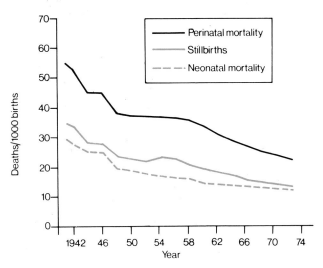

Figure 1. *Mortality trends in the UK, 1942–1972. The perinatal mortality and stillbirth rates are expressed as the number of deaths per thousand total births; the neonatal mortality rate is expressed as the number of deaths per thousand live births.*

Fetal Size and Growth

Serial estimation of fetal size provides valuable information concerning growth. The metabolic, and perhaps neuronal, concomitants of poor intrauterine growth render the fetus ill-equipped to tolerate asphyxial insults to which the fully-grown fetus may adapt. After delivery, the occurrence of hypoglycaemia and respiratory distress secondary to meconium aspiration highlights the continuum of morbidity in the poorly grown fetus.

Maternal Weight Gain

Maternal weight gain during pregnancy is only partly a reflection of fetal growth. Although there is an association between low maternal weight gain or a falling maternal weight and light-for-dates babies this observation would allow only a small fraction of fetuses with growth retardation to be detected.

Abdominal Examination

Serial abdominal examination, including measurements of the fundal height, in centimetres above the upper border of the symphysis pubis, detects changes in uterine

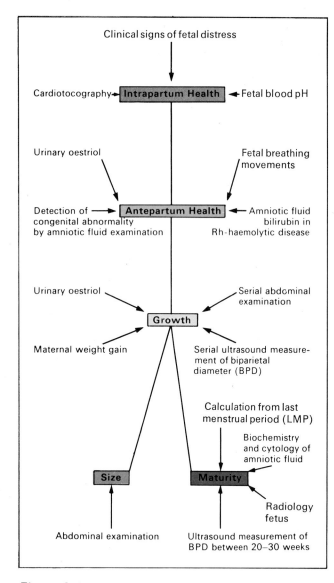

Figure 2. *Interrelation between fetal size, maturity, growth and health, and some methods of fetal assessment.*

Labels in figure:

Clinical signs of fetal distress

Cardiotocography → **Intrapartum Health** ← Fetal blood pH

Urinary oestriol

Fetal breathing movements

Detection of → **Antepartum Health** ← Amniotic fluid bilirubin in congenital abnormality by amniotic fluid examination — Rh-haemolytic disease

Urinary oestriol — Serial abdominal examination

Growth

Maternal weight gain — Serial ultrasound measurement of biparietal diameter (BPD)

Calculation from last menstrual period (LMP)

Biochemistry and cytology of amniotic fluid

Size — **Maturity**

Radiology fetus

Abdominal examination — Ultrasound measurement of BPD between 20–30 weeks

size. Uterine size is also influenced by amniotic fluid volume but this method of assessing fetal growth is not accurate enough to detect fetal growth retardation except in severe cases.

Measurement of Fetal Biparietal Diameter (BPD) by Ultrasonic Cephalometry

A narrow beam of ultrasound is projected at the fetal head through the maternal abdomen (Figure 3a). Some of the ultrasonic energy is reflected at each tissue interface. When the incident beam strikes a tissue interface at right-angles the echo returns along a reciprocal path to the source of production, which also acts as a receiving transducer and converts the returning echo into an electrical signal. In the single dimension A-scan the electrical signal appears as a series of deflections or 'blips' on a cathode ray oscilloscope (Figure 3b). The echo strength is proportional to the height of the deflection. The distance between the two strong echoes from either side of the fetal head at its widest diameter is proportional to the BPD. No complications from the use of diagnostic ultrasound have been reported in human fetuses.

Serial measurements of BPD reflect brain growth and, by implication, body growth. The normal mean weekly increment of BPD falls from 3.09 mm at 25 weeks to 1.23 mm at 39 weeks. Serial measurements may best be interpreted by plotting them on a graph which relates BPD to gestational age (Figure 4). The period of time which should elapse between scans before the growth rate can be reliably determined has yet to be firmly established. The brain is probably the last organ to be affected in fetal growth retardation; it would appear that a sub-normal rate of increase of the BPD reflects a fairly severe degree of fetal growth retardation.

Figure 3. a) *Measurement of fetal biparietal diameter by ultrasonic scanning;* **b)** *The scan readout. X represents midline structures of the fetal brain and AA represents the two parietal bones. The biparietal diameter is proportional to the distance A–A.*

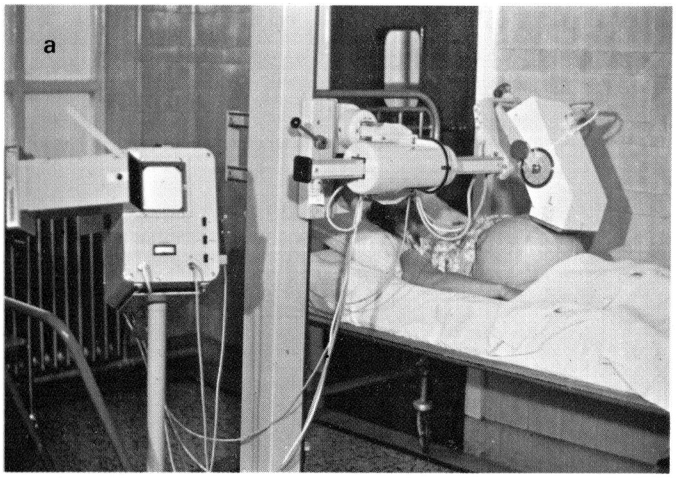

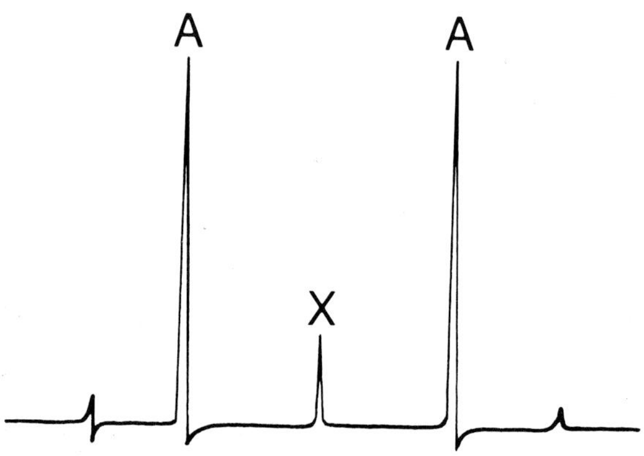

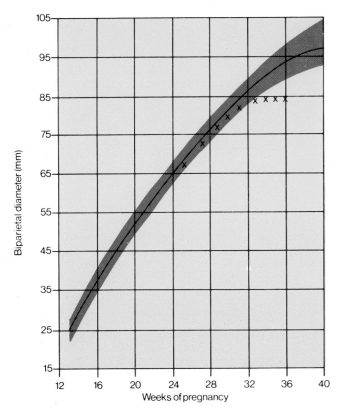

Figure 4. *The mean (± 2 SD) biparietal diameter at each gestational age (Campbell, 1969). Serial measurements of biparietal diameter (X) during pregnancy demonstrate failure of growth from 32 weeks.*

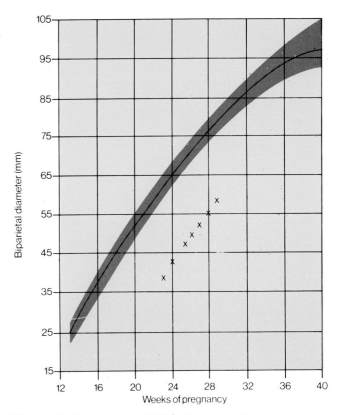

Figure 5. *The mean (± 2 SD) biparietal diameter at each gestational age (Campbell 1969). Serial measurements of biparietal diameter (X) during pregnancy suggest a normal rate of growth and an overestimation of the gestational age of the fetus by seven weeks.*

Fetal Maturity

The gestational age of the fetus is conventionally assessed from the date of the first day of the mother's last menstrual period (LMP). In early pregnancy the whole of the uterus can be examined bimanually and the experienced clinician can estimate the gestational age with considerable accuracy before the 12th week. All too often, particularly in pregnancies where the fetus is considered to be in jeopardy, the patient does not present to her doctor until the pregnancy is well-advanced and the LMP is not known with certainty.

Radiology

The appearance and size of the ossification centres of the fetus may be assessed by a plain X-ray of the maternal abdomen. The hazards of exposing the mother and fetus to a single X-ray are greatly outweighed by the diagnostic value of the information obtained. The time of appearance of certain ossification centres is shown in Table 1. In most cases bone maturity reflects the maturity of the fetus as a whole. However, discrepancies in the appearances of ossification centres have been noted in individual fetuses of twin pregnancies, and bone maturation in advance of gestational age has been reported in pregnancies complicated by maternal diabetes mellitus (Russell 1969). Growth retarded fetuses are a hetero-

genous group in terms of aetiology. It is possible that delayed bone maturation which is sometimes present is related to the cause of the growth retardation and is thereby a feature of some but not all 'light-for-dates' fetuses.

Ultrasonic Cephalometry

Attention has previously been drawn to the role of serial measurements of BPD by ultrasonics in the assessment of fetal growth. This method may also be used to assess fetal maturity if several measurements are made between 20 and 30 weeks gestation (Campbell 1969). During this period, growth of the fetal head is rapid and biological variation in BPD at each week of gestation is small (Figure 5).

Table 1. Time of appearance of ossification centres[1].

Talus	26 weeks
Calcaneum	28 weeks
Lower femur	37 weeks
Upper tibia	38 weeks

[1]Russell (1969)

3

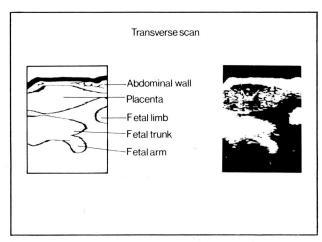

Figure 6. *Location of placental site by ultrasonic B-scan.*

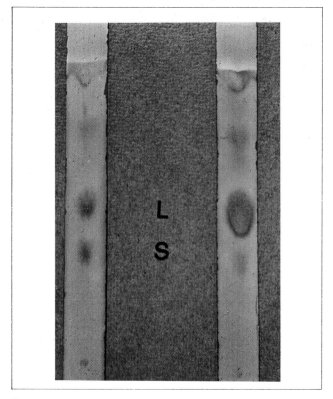

Figure 7. *A thin-layer chromatogram of amniotic fluid. The lecithin/sphingomyelin ratio (L/S) is determined by comparing the area of the lecithin spot (L) with the area of the sphingomyelin spot (S). The L/S ratio of the specimen on the right is greater than 2, whereas that on the left is less than 2.*

Amniocentesis

The biochemical and cytological composition of the amniotic fluid reflects fetal maturity. The placental site is located using the ultrasonic B-scan which provides a two-dimensional picture (Figure 6). A needle is inserted via the maternal abdomen through the uterus and into the amniotic cavity, avoiding the placental site; 5–10 ml of amniotic fluid are withdrawn. The risks involved in amniocentesis include fetal or maternal bleeding, blood group sensitisation and infection. Apparently 0.5 per cent of all amniocenteses are followed by spontaneous abortion, but amniocentesis is done for high risk pregnancies.

The Fetal Kidneys

These make an increasing contribution to the amniotic fluid in the latter half of pregnancy. After the first trimester there is a progressive fall in amniotic fluid osmolality and sodium concentration. After 30 weeks gestation the urea and creatinine concentrations rise steadily. The wide range in concentration of constituents at a given gestational age precludes the use of these measurements as a reliable indicator of gestational age.

Fetal Lung Fluid

This contains lecithin, a surface-active phospholipid which contributes to the amniotic fluid. A sharp increase in amniotic fluid lecithin concentration occurs at 34–36 weeks gestation in uncomplicated pregnancies. This signifies that sufficient surface-active material is present in the alveolar spaces to ensure their stability and prevent their collapse following the onset of respiration after birth. Premature delivery before a functional surface-active alveolar lining has developed is the single most important factor associated with the occurrence of idiopathic respiratory distress syndrome (IRDS) or hyaline membrane disease. When elective delivery before term is contemplated the measurement of amniotic fluid lecithin concentration can thus predict the major cause of mortality in babies born prematurely. IRDS is unlikely to occur if the pre-delivery result is above 3.5 mg per cent.

The rise in amniotic fluid lecithin concentration at 34–36 weeks is not matched by an increase in sphingomyelin which is a less important surface-active phospholipid. A technically simpler measurement is the lecithin: sphingomyelin (L/S) ratio by thin-layer chromatography (Figure 7). Whitfield (1973) reviewed a combined series of 1,049 pre-delivery L/S ratio estimates. When the ratio was below two, nearly 50 per cent of babies developed IRDS. In contrast, when the ratio was above two the incidence of IRDS was only two per cent. The fetal lung's acquisition of normal surface-active properties may occur quite suddenly in the space of a few days; measurements made one or two days before delivery have a greater predictive value than those made a week or more prior to delivery.

Desquamated Skin Cells

These appear in the amniotic fluid as the fetal skin matures. Cells derived from skin undergoing sebaceous activity contain lipid which stains orange with Nile blue sulphate. If 50 per cent or more of the cells stain orange it suggests that the fetus is at term or beyond. The converse does not apply and pregnancy at term may not be associated with the presence of orange-staining cells, thus limiting the role of this test in the assessment of fetal maturity.

Antepartum Fetal Health

Normal fetal growth is just one expression of fetal well-being; of the many other parameters of fetal health which have been studied, a few of current interest will be discussed.

Maternal Oestriol Excretion

The fetal adrenals produce dehydroepiandrosterone sulphate which is converted by the placenta to oestriol. The 24-hour maternal urinary oestriol excretion partly reflects the functional state of the placenta. Normal pregnancy is characterised by a rise in maternal oestriol excretion as gestation advances. The wide range of results for a given gestational age, and the considerable day-to-day variation in oestriol excretion, preclude the use of this measurement as an indicator of gestational age. A serial fall in 24-hour oestriol excretion suggests that the fetus is in jeopardy. As maternal urinary oestriol excretion partly reflects fetal adrenal activity, it is not surprising that abnormally low results occur in anencephaly with hypoplastic adrenal glands, or when fetal adrenal function is depressed by the administration of corticosteroids to the mother. Other drugs such as ampicillin, meprobamate (Equanil) and methenamine mandelate (Mandelamine) may lead to falsely low results.

Fetal Breathing Movements

Boddy and Robinson (1971) evolved a method of detecting breathing movements in human fetuses whereby a narrow beam of ultrasound is directed through the maternal abdomen and the echo from the fetal chest wall is identified and movements detected. Fetal breathing movements have been detected as early as 11 weeks gestation and occur from 55 to 90 per cent of the time. Although this method of assessing fetal health is a research tool at present, preliminary evidence suggests that the absence of normal fetal breathing and the presence of gasping movements indicate that the fetus is in jeopardy.

Amniotic Fluid Bilirubin in Rh Negative Haemolytic Disease

Care of the fetus with Rh negative haemolytic disease is directed towards preventing intrauterine death, and promoting the delivery of the baby in the best possible health. The mortality in babies who are born severely anaemic with gross oedema and heart failure is extremely high in spite of improved standards of resuscitation.

The Rh-antibody titre in maternal serum does not always correlate with the severity of the disease, and a more accurate assessment of the degree of fetal blood haemolysis is provided by the serial measurement of amniotic fluid bilirubin concentration by spectrophotometry. The maximum light absorption by bilirubin occurs at a wavelength of 450 nm. The difference between the actual optical density and a projected baseline reading at this wavelength is referred to as the optical density difference ($\triangle$OD) (see Figure 8a). The greater the $\triangle$OD, the higher the bilirubin concentration. A graph described by Liley (1961) relates $\triangle$OD to gestational age and is used in many maternity hospitals to assess the severity of the haemolytic process at a given gestational age (Figure 8b). Serial measurements of $\triangle$OD can detect the fetus who is becoming more severely affected as gestation advances and on these findings a decision may be made to deliver the fetus prematurely or perform an intrauterine transfusion.

Detection of Congenital Abnormalities by Amniotic Fluid Examination

The assessment of fetal health includes surveillance for

Figure 8a. *The measurement of amniotic fluid bilirubin by spectrophotometry. The optical density difference (ΔOD) of the specimen was 0.17.*
Figure 8b. *The ΔOD was plotted against gestational age (35 weeks) and the result suggested that the fetus was severely affected (•).*

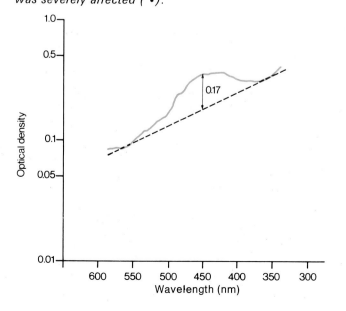

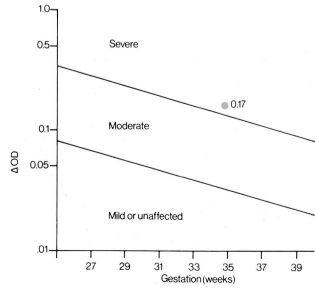

metabolic or structural abnormalities, some of which may now be suspected or diagnosed early in pregnancy. Amniotic fluid may be examined biochemically and cultured amniotic cells may be used for chromosome analysis or for the study of enzyme activity. This subject is discussed in Chapter 13.

Intrapartum Fetal Health

Abnormalities of fetal heart rate detected by intermittent auscultation and the presence of meconium-stained amniotic fluid are signs of fetal asphyxia. Fetal health may be compromised before such clinical signs are recognised, and the decision to expedite delivery may be made only after the fetus has suffered a lengthy period of asphyxia *in utero*. The improved accuracy with which fetal asphyxia in labour can now be recognised has been associated with a reduction in the Caesarean section rate for fetal distress (Beard 1968), and a fall in the perinatal mortality rate in some centres.

Cardiotocography

Continuous recordings of fetal heart rate may be made in conjunction with the measurement of intrauterine pressure changes.

Phonocardiography

A microphone applied to the maternal abdomen detects the fetal heart sounds which can be converted into an instantaneous rate reading.

Doppler Ultra-sound Cardiography

Ultrasound waves transmitted to the fetus via the maternal abdomen are reflected from the major fetal vessels. The frequency of the reflected sound waves varies with the movement of the reflecting structure (Doppler effect). The returning signal is transmitted as an amplified sound or recorded as an instantaneous rate (Figure 9).

Fetal Electrocardiography

Direct measurements of the fetal ECG may be obtained using an electrode passed through the cervix and clipped to the fetal scalp. The time interval between each 'R' wave is computed into an instantaneous rate recording.

Intrauterine pressure changes may be measured indirectly using a pressure sensitive device incorporated in a disc applied to the maternal abdomen. Direct measurements of intrauterine pressure are obtained by introducing into the amniotic cavity via the cervix a saline-filled catheter attached to a pressure transducer.

The Significance of Fetal Heart Rate Patterns

The normal fetal heart rate pattern is characterised by a rate of 120–160 per minute, no change in overall rate throughout the uterine contraction, and a 'beat to beat' variation of about eight beats per minute. Among the many fetal heart rate patterns which have been described, at least three have been shown to be associated

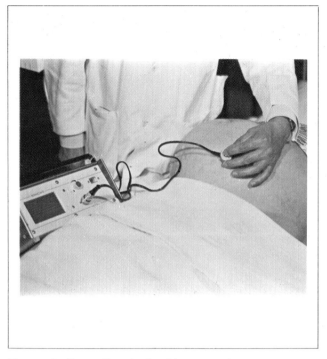

Figure 9. *Recording the fetal heart rate by Doppler ultrasound.*

with a greater incidence of fetal acidosis and delay in establishing normal respirations after birth compared with normal fetal heart rate patterns (Figure 10).

The Detection of Fetal Acidosis

The asphyxiated fetus depends upon anaerobic glycolysis for energy production. The accumulation of lactic and pyruvic acids leads to a metabolic acidosis. An amnioscope is passed through the cervix, and after removal of the obturator a stab incision is made in the fetal scalp. The blood (0.2–0.4 ml) is collected in a heparinised capillary tube and the pH is measured immediately. Generally a pH below 7.2 is considered abnormal. However up to 55 per cent of fetuses with a low pH show no clinical evidence of asphyxia at birth and, conversely, up to 15 per cent of fetuses with a normal pH show some clinical evidence of asphyxia at birth. Complications of this procedure include sepsis and sub-aponeurotic haemorrhage (Burke and Balfour 1976).

Treatment of the Unborn Baby

The well-established practice of maintaining maternal health during pregnancy forms the basis of providing the fetus with an optimal intrauterine environment. When fetal health is compromised by a poor environment, removal of the fetus from the hostile womb is one form of treatment. Occasionally it is possible to effect therapy by direct manipulation of the fetus or indirectly by drugs given to the mother.

Acceleration of Fetal Lung Maturation

Preliminary evidence suggests that the administration of the synthetic glucocorticoid betamethasone to pregnant

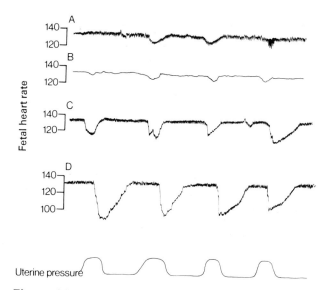

Figure 10. *Cardiotocography: four fetal heart rate patterns (A, B, C and D) are shown in association with uterine pressure changes during contractions.*

A: Normal; minimal cardiac slowing is seen with some contractions, and the amplitude of oscillation shows a 'beat to beat' variation of 5–8 per minute.

B: Loss of 'beat to beat' variation is shown by a grossly diminished amplitude of oscillation.

C: Variable dips; cardiac slowing shows a variable time relationship with uterine pressure. Note that the bradycardia associated with the uterine contraction on the extreme right persists beyond the end of the contraction.

D: Late dips: significant bradycardia persists beyond the end of each contraction.

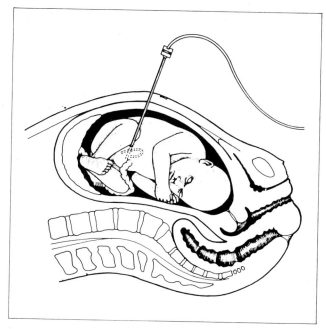

Figure 11. *Intrauterine transfusion for Rh-haemolytic disease. The blood is transfused via a catheter sited in the fetal peritoneal cavity.*

women is associated with a reduced incidence of IRDS in prematurely born babies (Liggins and Howie 1972). The drug probably acts by stimulating the enzymes responsible for lecithin production in the fetal lung. It is too early to assess the value of this drug but if proved efficacious its main use will be in pregnancies where premature labour if threatened, or when the clinician elects to deliver a baby prematurely because of poor fetal health.

Intrauterine Blood Transfusion

Occasionally the Rh-sensitised fetus is so severely affected by anaemia early in gestation that intrauterine death is imminent. When the fetus is so immature that elective delivery cannot be considered (less than 32–34 weeks), an intrauterine blood transfusion may be performed. Radiopaque dye is injected into the amniotic cavity 24 hours before the procedure so that the fetal skin and gastrointestinal tract are outlined on X-ray screening, thereby providing landmarks for the identification of the fetal peritoneal cavity. A needle through which polyethylene tubing is threaded is passed into the fetal peritoneal cavity via the maternal abdomen (Figure 11); 50–150 ml of packed red blood cells (O negative) are injected into the peritoneal cavity in 10 ml units over a period of two hours. Transfusion is generally required every seven to ten days until early delivery can be accomplished.

Conclusion

The clinician now has a considerable armament for the assessment of the unborn baby. Applying some of these newer techniques may not only make life more safe for the fetus, but should shed light on the complex interrelation between fetal size, maturity, growth and health.

References

Beard, R. W., *J. Obstet. Gynaec. Brit. Cwlth.*, 1968, **75**, 1291.
Boddy, K. and Robinson, J. S., *Lancet*, 1971, **ii**, 1231.
Burke, M. and Balfour, R., *Hosp. Update*, 1976, **2**, 237.
Campbell, S., *J. Obstet. Gynaec. Brit. Cwlth.*, 1969, **76**, 603.
Liggins, G. C. and Howie, R. N., *Pediatrics*, 1972, **50**, 515.
Liley, A. W., *Amer. J. Obstet. Gynec.*, 1961, **82**, 1359.
Russell, J. G. B., *J. Obstet. Gynaec. Brit. Cwlth.*, 1969, **76**, 208.
Whitfield, C. R., *Europ. J. Obstet. Gynec. Reprod. Biol.*, 1973, **3/6**, 215.

Further Reading

Symposium on Management of the High-Risk Pregnancy, *Clin. Perinatol.*, 1974, **1**, 185.
Steer, P. J., 1977, *Br. J. Hosp. Med.*, 1977, **17**, 219.

2. Cardiorespiratory and Thermal Adaptation to Extrauterine Life

ADAPTATION to extrauterine life involves functional modifications in virtually every organ-system of the body. Separation of the fetus from the placenta at birth is a dramatic milestone in the development of physiological processes related to gaseous exchange. No less an important event is separation of the fetus from the stable thermal environment of the uterus. The event of birth suddenly tests the integrity of cardiorespiratory and thermal homeostasis. Supportive care in the immediate newborn period should be based on an understanding of the pathophysiology of these homeostatic mechanisms.

Circulatory Adaptation

The Fetal Circulation

The placenta is the organ of gaseous exchange in fetal life. The circulation is modified to accommodate placental perfusion and is so designed that fetal arterial blood with the greatest oxygen content supplies the heart and brain, and less saturated blood passes to the lower part of the body and placenta (Figure 12).

Approximately 50 per cent of the umbilical venous blood ($Po_2 \simeq 40$ mm Hg) returning from the placenta bypasses the hepatic circulation and enters the inferior vena cava via the ductus venosus. Inferior vena caval blood divides into two streams so that 60 per cent passes directly into the left atrium through the foramen ovale and the remainder passes into the right atrium where it mixes with less saturated blood ($Po_2 \simeq 19$ mm Hg) returning from the head and neck in the superior vena cava. As a result, blood in the left ventricle is more saturated with oxygen than blood in the right ventricle. Left ventricular blood, which is approximately 60 per cent saturated with oxygen, is pumped into the ascending aorta and supplies the coronary arteries, cerebral circulation, head and neck, and upper extremities. Approximately 90 per cent of the blood ejected into the pulmonary artery from the right ventricle bypasses the lungs and enters the descending aorta via the ductus arteriosus. Blood in the descending aorta is thereby 'diluted' with blood of a lower oxygen saturation derived from the right ventricle; the resultant oxygen saturation is approximately 58 per cent.

Changes in the Circulation at Birth

A dramatic fall in pulmonary arteriolar resistance and increase in pulmonary blood flow occur when the lungs are ventilated at birth. The augmented pulmonary venous return to the left atrium is associated with a rise in left atrial pressure and functional closure of the flap-like valve of the foramen ovale. The fetal pulmonary–systemic pressure relationships are reversed and the systemic pressure becomes greater than the pulmonary pressure, leading to temporary left to right shunting through the ductus arteriosus. Constriction of the ductus arteriosus is brought about by the direct effect of the raised arterial Po_2 on the wall of the vessel. There is probably a rapid initial constriction soon after birth followed by a more gradual closure during the course of several days.

Circulatory adaptation to extrauterine life is not an event which is completed at once after birth; it is a dynamic process which may take hours or even days for completion. The pulmonary–systemic pressure relationship is largely dependent on the reactivity of the pulmonary vascular bed. Hypoxia and acidosis, features of many different cardiac and respiratory diseases of the newborn, cause pulmonary arteriolar vasoconstriction, pulmonary hypertension and reduced pulmonary blood flow. In these circumstances pulmonary venous return to the left atrium is reduced, left atrial pressure falls and right to left shunting of blood through the foramen ovale is facilitated. Pulmonary hypertension also encourages right to left shunting through the ductus arteriosus. The reactivity of the pulmonary vascular bed is an important phenomenon which influences the magnitude and direction of shunts through fetal channels in the transitional period after birth.

Respiratory Adaptation

During fetal life the lungs are fluid-filled, the volume being similar to the functional residual capacity after birth. An important biochemical constituent of lung fluid is lecithin, which has surface-active properties; hence its popular name, surfactant. When air is introduced into the lungs at birth, an air/liquid interface comprising surfactant forms the alveolar lining. The physical properties

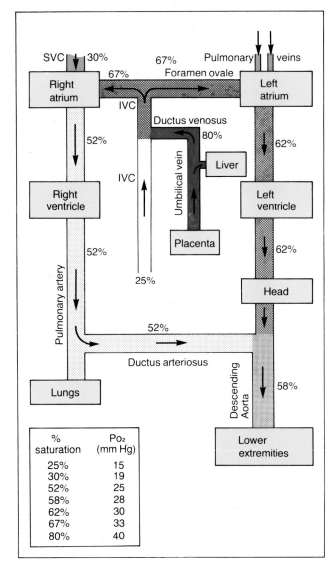

% saturation	P_{O_2} (mm Hg)
25%	15
30%	19
52%	25
58%	28
62%	30
67%	33
80%	40

Figure 12. *Diagram showing distribution of umbilical venous blood within the fetus, and the percentage oxygen saturation in different parts of the circulation.*

Table 2. Some causes of birth asphyxia.

1. Central

Respiratory depression:
Prolonged fetal asphyxia in labour
Sedative/analgesic drugs administered to mother during labour.
Trauma to brain stem:
Haemorrhage
Herniation

2. Peripheral

Airway obstruction
Congenital malformations of respiratory tract:
Pulmonary hypoplasia
Diaphragmatic hernia
Thoracic dystrophy

Table 3. Apgar score[1].

Sign	Score		
	0	1	2
Heart rate	Absent	< 100	> 100
Respiratory effort	Absent	Weak Gasping Irregular	Good Crying Regular
Muscle tone	Completely flaccid	Some flexion of extremities	Well flexed
Reflex irritability, e.g. response to nasal catheter	No response	Grimace	Cough Sneeze Gasp
Colour of trunk	White	Blue	Pink

[1]Apgar, 1953

of the surfactant lining are such that the surface tension effect at the air/liquid interface is minimised, facilitating alveolar expansion and stabilising and preventing the collapse of small alveoli.

The control mechanisms responsible for the transition from fetal 'respiratory' activity to normal ventilation at birth are a subject of continual debate. It is enough to say that the transition is triggered by tactile and thermal stimuli and that in addition central chemosensory mechanisms have been shown to be operative in fetal and neonatal life. A negative intrathoracic pressure of up to 100 cm H_2O has been recorded during the first breath, which has a volume of about 30–40 ml. Lung compliance increases within the first few hours of life and a normal tidal volume of 20–30 ml, requiring a negative intrathoracic pressure of 5 cm H_2O, is established. The clearance of fetal lung fluid occurs via the mouth, aided by the effect of thoracic compression within the birth canal. Lung fluid is also absorbed into the pulmonary lymphatics.

The Pathophysiology of Birth Asphyxia

Failure to establish normal respiration soon after birth is associated with the biochemical changes of hypoxaemia, hypercapnia, and acidaemia. The causes may be conveniently divided into central and peripheral (Table 2). Central causes are more common, particularly reduced 'respiratory drive' due to sedative or analgesic drugs administered to the mother during labour, or fetal asphyxia in labour.

The severity of birth asphyxia is commonly measured by the Apgar score, a clinical assessment based on the evaluation of five physical signs (Table 3). When the Apgar score is accurately assessed and recorded by an experienced observer it can provide information which may be useful in retrospect. In this context the score measured at five minutes after birth is more relevant than the one minute score. Obsession with Apgar scoring as a nursing administrative procedure has perhaps focused attention away from the real problem, i.e. the rational management of the asphyxiated baby, based on an understanding of the pathophysiology of the condition.

Events associated with birth asphyxia in man are probably similar to those described in the rhesus monkey following experimentally induced total asphyxia at birth (Dawes 1968) (Figure 13). Soon after the onset of the asphyxial insult rapid gasps occur which cease after about a minute. This is followed by a period of 'primary apnoea'. Spontaneous deep gasping follows for several minutes, gradually becoming weaker and terminating in the 'last gasp'. The time interval between the asphyxial insult and the last gasp is about eight minutes. 'Terminal apnoea' follows the last gasp unless resuscitation is started.

In man, the occurrence of a sudden complete asphyxial insult at birth is rare; intermittent partial asphyxia during labour is more common. Most babies are born in primary apnoea and rapidly establish normal respiration.

Primary Apnoea

The clinical features of primary apnoea are shown in Table 4. During the early stages the blood pressure is normal or may be raised. Maintenance of the circulation under hypoxic conditions is partly due to the high concentration of cardiac glycogen which acts as a substrate for anaerobic glycolysis. An oxygen conserving mechanism operates whereby blood is preferentially directed to the brain, heart and adrenal glands. The intimate relationship between circulatory and respiratory events at birth is illustrated in the asphyxial situation. Hypoxaemia, acidaemia and failure of lung expansion are associated with pulmonary hypertension, and the persistence of certain fetal circulatory characteristics is a feature of birth asphyxia.

Terminal Apnoea

An asphyxiated baby may make a few weak gasps following a period of primary apnoea and enter the stage of terminal apnoea. Alternatively, a baby may be born in terminal apnoea having gone through the gasping stage *in utero*. The clinical features of terminal apnoea are shown in Table 4. Circulatory failure and hypotension, which are prominent features at this stage, are probably largely due to a depletion of cardiac glycogen stores.

Some Practical Implications

A paediatrician should be present at the delivery in circumstances where there is an increased risk of birth asphyxia (Table 5).

In primary apnoea various stimuli such as a gentle slap on the soles of the feet usually induce a gasp or cry. Unduly painful stimulation is unnecessary and cruel. Gasping occurs in response to pharyngeal suction. Oxygen, administered by a face mask, will not reach the lungs if the baby is apnoeic, but gasping is usually induced because of the stimulatory effect of the flow of cold gas over the facial skin. When oxygen is administered by

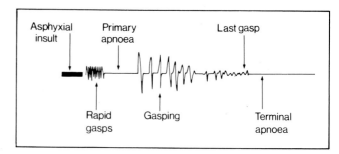

Figure 13. *The sequence of respiratory events that occurs following the application of an asphyxial insult to a rhesus monkey at birth.*

Table 4. Clinical features of primary and terminal apnoea.

Primary apnoea

Heart rate > 100, accelerating
Blood pressure normal or raised
Colour of trunk blue rather than white
Small spontaneous movement often seen, e.g. lips, eyelids
Some flexion of extremities
Reflex response to manipulation, e.g. gasps or coughs in response to nasal catheter.

Terminal apnoea

Heart rate < 100, slowing
Hypotension
Colour of trunk white
No spontaneous movements seen
Completely flaccid extremities
No reflex response to manipulation

Table 5. Indications for alerting the paediatrician to be present at delivery.

Evidence of fetal asphyxia
Caesarean section
Dystocia
Abnormal presentation
Large dose of sedative/analgesic drugs administered to mother late in labour
Abruptio placentae, placenta praevia
Rupture of membranes > 24 hours
Multiple pregnancy
Prematurity
Gestation > 42 weeks
Intrauterine growth retardation
Toxaemia
Diabetes mellitus
Erythroblastosis fetalis
Elderly primigravida

intermittent positive pressure ventilation (IPPV) via a face mask and bag, initial expansion of the lungs induces a reflex gasp. This is known as Head's paradoxical reflex. Certain analgesics such as pethidine and morphine given to the mother late in labour prolong the stage of primary apnoea; in these circumstances nalorphine (0.1 to 0.2 mg/kg) or naloxone HCl (0.01 mg/kg) may be given via the umbilical vein. There is no indication for the use of analeptic drugs in the management of birth asphyxia.

In terminal apnoea or gasping associated with a falling heart rate some form of IPPV is mandatory and takes priority over all other procedures. Following intubation, IPPV may be given by the manual squeezing of an oxygen-filled bag, by mechanical ventilation or, as is usual in hospital practice by the use of an intermittent occlusion device (Figure 14). Mouth to mouth ventilation, or a face mask and bag apparatus, may be used when intubation is not feasible. Perfusion of vital organs is improved by external cardiac massage if the heart rate does not increase with IPPV. Acidaemia which is a feature of terminal apnoea may be treated by the intravenous administration of 8.4 per cent sodium bicarbonate (3 ml per kg bodyweight). The following sequence of events occurs following successful resuscitation:

1. Increase in heart rate.

2. Increase in blood pressure.

3. Pink coloration of skin.

4. Spontaneous gasping followed by normal respiration.

5. Return of spinal reflexes.

6. Return of muscle tone.

The Outcome Following Birth Asphyxia

It is indisputable that severe and prolonged birth asphyxia may cause brain damage. Bilateral, symmetrical lesions of the inferior colliculus, brain stem, cerebellum and thalamus were described in rhesus monkeys when the duration of the asphyxial insult exceeded the time to the last gasp (Ranck and Windle 1959). It was rare for the cerebral cortex to be involved. Evidence relating the birth asphyxia in man to brain damage is based on clinical studies. There are many pitfalls in this type of approach, not the least being the selection of criteria for establishing the occurrence and severity of birth asphyxia. Using the Apgar scoring system as a means of assessing the severity of asphyxia, it was demonstrated that of infants with a five minute score of 0 or 1, 44 per cent did not survive the second day of life, and approximately 50 per cent did not survive the first four weeks (Drage and Berendes 1966). Neurological abnormality at the age of one year was three times more common in infants who had an Apgar score of 0 – 3 than in those who had a score of 7–10.

Although it is comparatively simple to diagnose clinically severe forms of cerebral palsy and intellectual retardation, it is much more difficult to establish meaningful clinical criteria for recognising minor abnormalities of function and intellect. There is no sharp division between

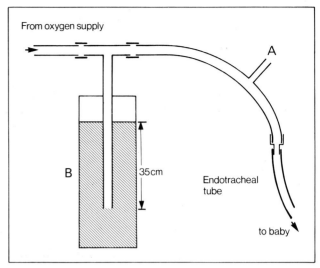

Figure 14. *Diagram of apparatus for giving intermittent positive pressure ventilation to babies at birth. The hole in the tubing (A) is intermittently occluded by the operator's finger. The water manometer (B) acts as a blow-off valve and prevents inflation pressures exceeding 35 cm H$_2$O.*

normality and abnormality in this respect.

An association between birth asphyxia and clinical evidence of brain damage at some time after birth does not necessarily imply a simple cause and effect phenomenon. The low birthweight baby who is prone to birth asphyxia is also vulnerable to a host of other afflictions which may influence the long-term outcome. There is also no doubt that given an asphyxial insult, acting alone or in combination with other pathology, the functional and intellectual outcome in later life is very powerfully influenced by the environmental framework that surrounds the individual's growth and development.

The parents of a baby who has suffered birth asphyxia invariably question what the future will hold for their baby. It is not uncommon for such a baby to demonstrate grossly abnormal neurological signs in the first few days of life, and for the signs to abate gradually over the next few days with apparently normal development ensuing. A poor prognosis should never be given unless there are very compelling reasons for doing so. The parent–baby bond in the first weeks of life may be adversely influenced by a few badly chosen words. It is prudent to admit uncertainty, and to stress the importance of repeated developmental assessment so that the picture of normality or abnormality has time to unfold gradually. As a general guide the following features have been shown to influence adversely the prognosis:

1. The occurrence of terminal rather than primary apnoea.

2. The presence of associated factors, particularly low birthweight and hypoglycaemia.

3. Frequent convulsions during the first few days of life.

4. The persistence of abnormal neurological signs.

5. Social deprivation of the family.

Thermal Adaptation to Extrauterine Life

The core temperature of the fetus is about 1°C higher than that of the mother, and one function of the placenta is the dissipation of heat produced by the fetus. After birth, the baby behaves as a homeotherm and brings into play mechanisms which allow the body temperature to be maintained at a fairly constant level despite fluctuations in the environmental temperature. Certain limitations are imposed on these adaptive mechanisms, particularly if the baby is of low birthweight.

In a given period of time, heat produced as a result of metabolic processes must equal heat losses if the body temperature is to remain constant. Shivering is not a feature of the newborn's response to a cool environment, although babies exposed to such an environment do exhibit an increase in physical activity. The newborn increases heat production by non-shivering thermogenesis in the face of cold stress. This adaptive mechanism is brought about by the metabolism of brown fat which is situated at the base of the neck, between the scapulae and surrounding the kidneys and adrenals. Brown fat accounts for two to six per cent of the total body weight of the newborn.

Heat loss from within the body to the body surface is regulated by changes in skin blood flow. Heat loss from the surface of the body to the environment occurs by the following mechanisms:

1. Radiation.

2. Convection.

3. Conduction.

4. Evaporation.

The contribution of each component varies considerably with different nursing conditions, being dependent on factors such as whether the baby is clothed or naked, the temperature gradient between the baby's skin and the nearest surface, the air speed, the nature of the surface, (e.g. mattress) in contact with the baby, and the water vapour pressure.

The Environmental Temperature

The normal adult can voluntarily modify the effect of a cool environment and thereby prevent heat loss: he may move to a warmer room or wear extra clothing. The newborn is dependent on his care-giver to provide the optimal thermal environment. There can be no doubt that the improved survival of low birthweight babies during the past 20–30 years is partly attributable to better standards of nursing care based on insight into the pathophysiology of thermal control.

The thermoneutral range for a given baby is the environmental temperature range at which oxygen con-

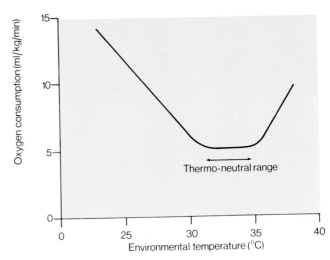

Figure 15. *Relationship between oxygen consumption of the newborn and environmental temperature (Hill 1959).*

Table 6. The thermoneutral range (°C) on day 1 and day 10 in babies of 1.0 kg, 2.0 kg, and 3.0 kg birthweight nursed naked or clothed.[1]

	Day 1	Day 10
1.0 kg		
Unclothed	34.5 – 35.5	33.0 – 34.5
Clothed	28.5 – 31.0	26.0 – 29.0
2.0 kg		
Unclothed	33.0 – 34 5	31.0 – 34.0
Clothed	25.0 – 29.5	21.0 – 27.0
3.0 kg		
Unclothed	32.0 – 34.0	30.5 – 33.5
Clothed	23.0 – 29.0	20.0 – 26.5

Unclothed babies were nursed in an incubator with a perspex heat shield in position. Clothed babies were nursed in a cot with light blankets.

[1] Hey and Katz (1970)

sumption is minimal in the presence of a normal body temperature. The relationship between oxygen consumption and environmental temperature is shown in Figure 15. The thermoneutral range varies under different nursing conditions, e.g. whether the baby is naked or clothed, and is influenced by body weight and postnatal age (Table 6). A baby nursed below the thermoneutral range responds by increasing heat production and thereby oxygen consumption. A normal central body temperature is achieved at a caloric cost, valuable calories being diverted from the maintenance of growth. A normal body temperature (rectal 37°C) does not necessarily imply that the baby is being nursed in the optimal thermal environment. A subnormal body temperature indicates that the homeothermic processes have been overwhelmed. If the environment is above the thermoneutral range, hyperthermia may rapidly develop. It is significant that the newborn, particularly the small pre-term baby, does not sweat effectively.

Figure 16. *Top: Baby nursed in incubator which has an air temperature of 33°C. The room temperature is cool (19°C), and consequently the inside wall of the incubator falls to 28°C, provoking significant radiant heat loss from the baby (straight arrows). Bottom: a perspex heat shield is interposed between the baby and the wall of the incubator. The temperature of the inside wall of the heat shield is similar to the incubator air temperature (33°C) and radiant heat loss from the baby is minimised.*

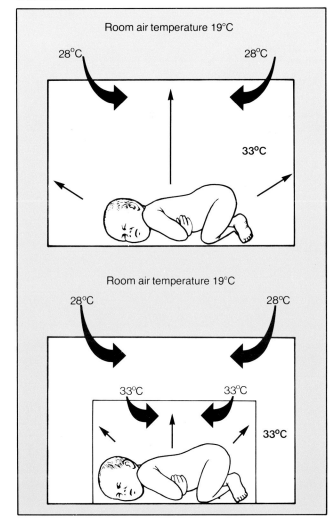

Some Practical Implications

A baby is especially at risk of developing a subnormal body temperature, because of undue heat loss, in certain situations.

At birth the baby is naked and wet. A delivery-room temperature that is comfortable for the mother and mid-wife may be too cold for the baby. Evaporative heat loss may be minimised by gently drying the baby soon after birth. Unless the clinical situation warrants close observation the baby should be clothed immediately.

The other situations where the baby may be naked and exposed to an ambient temperature below the neutral range are during clinical examination, investigative procedures, e.g. X-ray, surgical procedures, and at bath time.

Transporting a newborn baby from home to hospital, or between different hospitals, has many important nursing and medical implications; not the least is the provision of an optimal thermal environment during the journey, by the use of an efficient portable incubator.

A naked baby nursed in an incubator presents special problems. There will be a considerable loss of radiant heat from the baby if the temperature of the inside wall of the incubator is very much lower than that of the baby's skin. This situation occurs when the incubator is in a cool room. Radiant heat loss can be minimised by interposing a plastic shield between the baby and the inside wall of the incubator (Figure 16). Evaporative heat loss is minimised if the water vapour pressure, and hence the relative humidity, within the incubator is high. However, this advantage may be outweighed by the fact that a moist environment favours the growth of certain bacterial organisms, particularly *Pseudomonas*.

References

Apgar, V., *Anesth. Analg.,* 1953, **32,** 260.

Dawes, G. S., *Fetal and Neonatal Physiology,* Year Book Medical Publishers Inc., Chicago, 1968.

Drage, J. and Berendes, H., *Pediat. Clin. N. Amer.,* 1966, **13,** 635.

Hey, E. and Katz, G., *Arch. Dis. Child.,* 1970, **45,** 328.

Hill, J., *J. Physiol.,* 1959, **149,** 346.

Ranck, J., Jr. and Windle, W., *Exp. Neurol.,* 1959, **1,** 130.

Further Reading

Alexander, G., *Br. Med. Bull.,* 1975, **31,** 62.

Chernick, V. (Ed.), Onset and control of fetal and neonatal respiration. In *Seminars in Perinatology,* 1977, **1,** 321–383, Grune and Stratton, New York.

Hey, E., *Br. Med. Bull.,* 1975, **31,** 69.

Scott, H., *Arch. Dis. Childh.,* 1976, **51,** 712.

3. Examination of the Newborn

THE newborn baby should be examined within 24 hours of birth and again during the second week of life or just before discharge from the maternity hospital. The purposes of the initial examination are:

1. To detect certain congenital malformations which may be an immediate threat to life or which may need treatment later.

2. To detect illnesses which have arisen from an adverse intrauterine environment in the antenatal or intrapartum period (for example, intrauterine infection, haemolytic disease, birth asphyxia, birth trauma).

3. To measure and document parameters of body size.

4. To provide an opportunity for the mother to ask questions about her baby's appearance, such as the significance of minor skin blemishes.

The second examination is necessary to detect congenital malformations which may have been inapparent at birth and to detect newly acquired disease, the most common being infection. It also enables the baby's progress from birth to be assessed and provides an opportunity to answer the mother's questions about feeding, weight, behaviour, etc.

The examination should be carried out in the mother's presence and in a room which is suitably warm and well lit by natural daylight. It is prudent to avoid examination during the mother's mealtime, immediately before or soon after the baby has been fed, or when the baby has to be wakened from a deep sleep. Unclothing the baby is an integral part of the examination and is therefore the task of the doctor and not the nurse. The examination should combine brevity with a methodical approach and the scheme outlined in Table 7 is recommended.

General Observations

The Breathing Pattern

This should be assessed early in the examination before the baby has become too disturbed. Observe the alae nasi for flaring and listen for inspiratory stridor or expiratory grunting or whining. Gently lift the baby's vest and observe the chest wall for symmetry of movement, and signs of intercostal, subcostal or sternal recession on inspiration. The respiratory rate should be less than 60 per minute at rest.

Table 7. Examination of the newborn.

General observations:
    a) Breathing pattern
    b) Neurological behaviour
    c) Skin
Cranial vault
Face
Chest
Abdomen
Groin and genital region
Spine
Limbs
Parameters of body size

Neurological Behaviour

The normal full-term baby in the supine position lies with the limbs partially flexed, whereas the hypotonic baby tends to adopt a frog-like position of the lower limbs with the arms out-stretched alongside the trunk. When unclothing the baby pay particular attention to the resistance offered to this manoeuvre. The hypotonic baby offers little or no resistance and may behave rather like a rag-doll. In contrast, most normal babies resent being unclothed and their reluctance to part with their vest and napkin should not lead to a diagnosis of hypertonia. Observe for asymmetry of limb movements and remember that if this is present the cause may lie outside the nervous system (for example, fracture or osteitis). Attention should be given to the baby's cry and general demeanour throughout the examination. Provided that the examination has not been wrongly timed to occur immediately before or soon after a feed the following should arouse suspicion:

1. A baby who is lethargic and never cries throughout the examination.

2. A baby who resents every manoeuvre and who has a shrill high-pitched cry.

A more extensive neurological examination is necessary only if there is doubt about the normality of the baby's behaviour.

The Skin

The normal full-term baby is a healthy pale pink colour.

The unclothed baby should be carefully observed for pallor, plethora, cyanosis, jaundice and skin blemishes.

Pallor

The causes are anaemia due to haemorrhage or haemolytic disease and 'neurological shock' which is usually the result of birth asphyxia or birth trauma. The baby who is anaemic because of haemorrhage usually has an associated tachycardia. In anaemia caused by haemolysis, associated physical signs which should be looked for include jaundice and hepatosplenomegaly. The pallor associated with the 'neurological shock' of birth asphyxia or birth trauma is often associated with bradycardia, abnormal neurological signs, a history of fetal distress or a difficult manipulative delivery. Intracranial bleeding may co-exist.

Plethora

The very premature baby often has dark red skin, but in the full-term baby plethora may be caused by polycythaemia, extreme hypothermia or hyperthermia. Polycythaemia, which can be defined as a packed cell volume greater than 70 per cent, may be caused by maternofetal transfusion, fetofetal transfusion in the case of multiple pregnancy, or delayed clamping of the umbilical cord. The complications of neonatal polycythaemia include arterial and venous thrombosis and hyperbilirubinaemia. Extreme hypothermia and hyperthermia are more likely to be seen in domiciliary practice.

Jaundice

Neonatal jaundice is fully discussed in Chapter 7, but the following guide may be of help when examining the baby:

1. The presence of jaundice in the first 24 hours of life is always abnormal and is invariably caused by haemolytic disease. Jaundice detected at the subsequent examination *may* be 'physiological'.

2. The normal pink colour of the baby's skin may mask the presence of jaundice. Blanch the skin (for example, over the tip of the nose) by applying gentle pressure with the finger for a few seconds, and immediately assess the degree of jaundice when the finger is released.

3. When the bilirubin level is progressively increasing it is usual for the degree of jaundice to be clinically underestimated. Conversely, when the bilirubin level is falling it is usual to overestimate the degree of jaundice.

4. It is easy to underestimate grossly the degree of jaundice in African or Asiatic babies.

5. The degree of jaundice is usually underestimated in a baby receiving phototherapy. The light leaches the yellow from the skin and the serum bilirubin level is usually greater than one would expect.

Cyanosis

Blue discoloration of the extremities is common in the first few hours of life and soon disappears. Peripheral cyanosis in an otherwise well baby with a normal body temperature is of little significance. In contrast, central cyanosis is observed best in the tongue and inside of the lips and is always of serious consequence, denoting respiratory or cardiovascular disease. 'Traumatic cyanosis' is the name given to petechiae confined to the head and neck which give an overall blue appearance to that region. It should not be confused with central cyanosis as the pink tongue contrasts markedly against the blue face. 'Traumatic cyanosis' may occur if the cord has been stretched round the neck, or in face or brow presentation. In many cases there is no discernible cause. The condition clears spontaneously in a week or two and the mother should be told of the good prognosis.

Skin Blemishes

Most of the skin blemishes that are commonly seen in the newborn period fade spontaneously but they may sometimes be the source of considerable parental anxiety. Examination of the baby in the mother's presence provides an opportunity for her to ask questions about these lesions.

1. *Stork bites* (macular haemangiomata) are present in 30 to 50 per cent of newborn infants (Solomon and Esterly 1973). The common sites of involvement are the nape of the neck, the eyelids and the glabella. Most of these lesions fade spontaneously. Larger nuchal lesions may persist but they are rarely noticeable.

2. *Erythema toxicum* affects 30 to 70 per cent of newborn infants (Harris and Schick 1956; Taylor and Bondurant 1957) (Figure 17). The peak incidence is between 24 and 48 hours. The lesions, which fade spontaneously in a few days, consist of white papules (1 to 3 mm diameter) on an erythematous base. In some cases only the erythematous base is present. Any part of the skin may be involved except the palms and soles. The cause of the rash is unknown.

3. *Mongolian spot* is present in 90 per cent of Blacks and Orientals and in one to five per cent of Caucasian babies (Pratt 1953) (Figure 18). The most common sites of involvement are the lumbosacral region and the buttocks.

Figure 17. *Erythema toxicum.*

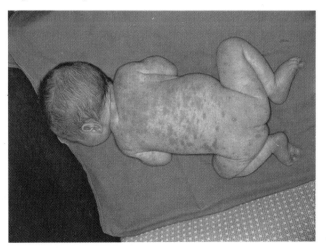

The lesions consist of single or multiple slate blue or grey macules, and usually fade within the first two years.

4. *Milia* are small epidermal cysts containing keratinous material which develop in connection with the pilo-sebaceous follicle. They affect 40 per cent of full-term infants and appear as pearly white or yellow papules (1 mm diameter) scattered over the cheeks, nose, and forehead. They disappear in the first few weeks of life.

5. *Sebaceous gland hyperplasia* is manifest as a myriad of minute white or yellow spots on the nose, upper lip and malar region. They are apparently not evident in pre-term babies (Solomon and Esterly 1973), and fade spontaneously in a few weeks.

6. *Port-wine stain* (*naevus flammeus*) is present at birth and is a permanent developmental dilatation of capillaries without endothelial proliferation (Figure 19). The lesion increases in size after birth in proportion to growth of the infant. Individual lesions, which are flat and pale pink to deep purple, vary enormously in size from baby to baby and may be situated anywhere on the skin, although facial lesions are the most common. Some lesions have a unilateral distribution.

7. *Strawberry naevus* is generally not apparent at birth but in most cases is evident by the second month of life. It is a raised capillary or cavernous haemangioma, which usually appears as a single lesion and most commonly affects the face, back, scalp or anterior chest wall. Most of these lesions increase in size in the first six months and regress completely by seven years of age.

The Cranial Vault

The size of the fontanelles and the degree of separation of the cranial sutures are usually of little significance provided that the occipitofrontal head circumference is appropriate for the baby's gestational age, the anterior fontanelle is not tense, and there are no abnormal neurological signs or symptoms. In the first few days of life overriding of the cranial sutures is a common finding in babies born by the vaginal route.

A cephalhaematoma is a swelling caused by bleeding under the periosteum of one or more of the cranial vault bones, usually the parietal bone. The swelling is bounded by sutures and becomes apparent during the second or third day of life. The breakdown of red blood corpuscles within the haematoma often leads to the development of mild jaundice. The mother should be warned that it may take weeks or months before the swelling disappears.

A caput succedaneum is an oedematous swelling of the presenting part caused by the constricting rim of the cervix obstructing venous and lymphatic return from the scalp. In contrast to the cephalhaematoma, the caput succedaneum overlies suture lines. It is present at birth and disappears after a few days.

Examination of the vault is not complete without careful observation along the midline area between the root of the nose and base of the skull in the occipital region. An encephalocele will usually be obvious but a congenital dermal sinus in this region often goes unnoticed.

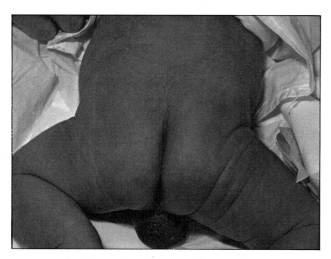

Figure 18. *Mongolian blue spots in a black baby.*

Figure 19. *Port-wine stain (naevus flammeus).*

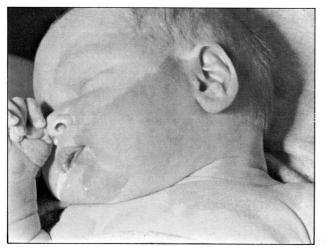

The Face

It is sometimes suspected that the baby has an odd-looking face. An attempt should be made to ascertain carefully and document any unusual characteristics which contribute to the composite facial appearance. Remember that crumpled ears and swollen eyelids are frequent findings soon after delivery. The most common abnormality which presents with an unusual facial appearance is Down's syndrome. Such babies are invariably hypotonic and have many clearly defined individual features of the condition such as an abnormal slant of the palpebral fissures, epicanthic folds and a small mouth. Most babies whose sole abnormality is said to be an odd-looking face have the facial characteristics of one or other of the parents and the mother will often volunteer gleefully that her baby 'looks just like his dad'.

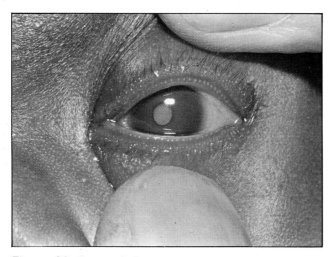

Figure 20. *Congenital cataract.*

Figure 21. *Cloudy cornea, a feature of congenital glaucoma.*

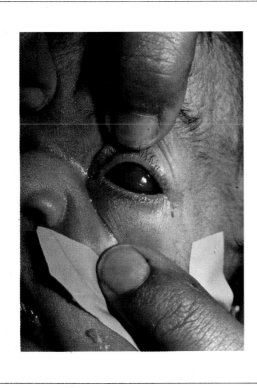

Points to be Observed

The eyelids should be held open gently while observing for:

1. Cataract which is best seen by shining a light obliquely into the eye (Figure 20).

2. Coloboma which appears as a sector-shaped gap in the iris.

3. Glaucoma which presents with a hazy cornea, increased intraocular tension and photophobia (Figure 21).

4. Subconjunctival haemorrhages which may be seen adjacent to the iris. They are harmless and disappear in a few weeks.

5. Conjunctivitis. Remember that a profuse purulent discharge from one or both eyes on the first day of life is likely to be caused by gonococcal infection.

The mouth should be clearly visualised with a bright torch. A large cleft palate is easily recognised but a small cleft in the soft palate may go unnoticed.

1. Epstein's pearls (epithelial pearls) occur in 85 per cent of newborn infants and are discrete round pearly structures located alongside the midline of the palate. They are the intraoral conterpart of facial milia and disappear during the first few weeks of life.

2. Natal teeth are occasionally seen in the incisor region. The dentist should be asked to remove these because of the risk of spontaneous exfoliation and aspiration. Such teeth are usually from the deciduous dentition (Figure 22).

3. A ranula is a mucous cyst which occurs in the floor of the mouth or beneath the tongue in relation to the submandibular or sublingual salivary ducts. Large ones may require surgical removal but smaller ones usually disappear spontaneously.

4. A short lingual frenulum is common and does not interfere with sucking or speech development.

5. Oral thrush situated on the tongue may be distinguished from a milk curd plaque by the fact that the former leaves a raw area when scraped.

Chest

Breast engorgement is common and harmless. It should not be confused with a breast abscess where the skin surrounding the breast tissue is inflamed. In the absence of signs of respiratory distress, listening to the breath sounds is of little value and should be omitted. A faint heart murmur heard during the initial examination in a well baby is likely to be innocent and disappear in a few days. It is unwise to draw the mother's attention to this finding. If the murmur does not disappear, or if a murmur is heard in a well baby for the first time before the discharge examination, the mother should be told of its existence. The baby should be reviewed later.

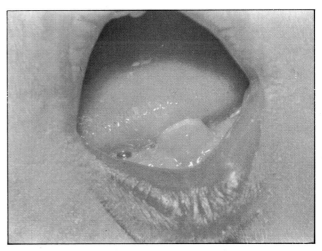

Figure 22. *Natal incisor tooth.*

Abdomen

Observe for abdominal distension. Examine the umbilicus for signs of sepsis or herniation of a viscus or omentum into the cord (Figure 23). If there is only one umbilical artery there is a greater chance that the baby has some other congenital abnormality. Palpate the abdomen for enlarged viscera. The liver edge is easy to feel 1 to 2 cm below the costal margin. Both kidneys are palpable; the spleen is just palpable in ten per cent of apparently normal neonates.

Groin and Genital Region

There are a number of important observations related to different organ systems which are conveniently grouped together in this region. Feel for a hernia in the groin, scrotum or labia. Ensure that the femoral pulse is present. Observe that an anal opening is present.

In the Male

Bruising of the scrotum is a common finding after breech delivery, and soon disappears (Figure 24). Ascertain the following points:

1. Is the prepuce hooded?
2. Is there hypospadias?
3. Are both testes in the scrotum?
4. Is there a hydrocele?

In the Female

Mucoid vaginal discharge is normal and it is not uncommon for menstruation lasting a few days to occur in the first week of life. The following points should be ascertained:

1. Are the labia fused?
2. Is the clitoris enlarged?

Figure 23. *Remnant of the distal portion of the omphalomesenteric duct presenting as a bright red umbilical polyp at the cut end of the cord.*

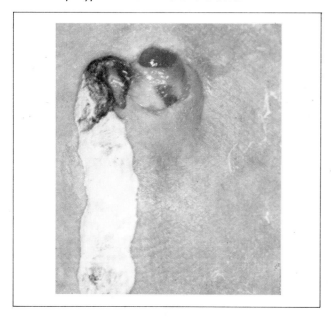

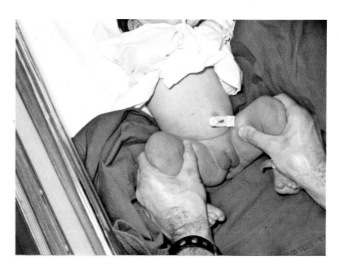

Figure 25. *Examining for congenital dislocation of the left hip. Above: first movement, adduction with lateral pressure exerted by the thumb. Simultaneously, downward pressure is exerted along the line of the thigh. Below: second movement, abduction with medial pressure exerted by the middle finger.*

Figure 24. *Bruised scrotum following breech delivery.*

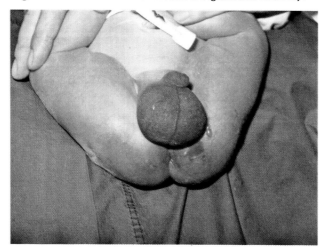

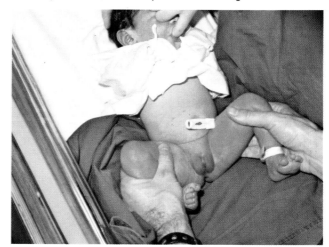

Spine

Examine the whole length of the spine most carefully. The presence of a myelomeningocele will be obvious. A midline hairy patch or naevus may be associated with an underlying spinal lesion such as spina bifida occulta or more rarely distematomyelia or an intradural lipoma. An x-ray of the spine should be performed during the first few months of life, and neurological examination of the limbs and appraisal of bladder and anal sphincter function once or twice during the first year. It is unnecessary to follow up babies with spina bifida occulta and it often provokes parental anxiety. A pit, several millimetres deep, in the sacrococcygeal region is a common finding. By gently retracting the skin at the margins of the pit a blind end can usually be seen. These pits are harmless. A pit above the level of S_2 usually communicates with the theca and the baby should be referred to a neurosurgeon as soon as possible because of the risk of meningitis.

Limbs

The hands may be easily overlooked if the fists are tightly clenched or if the doctor fails to remove the baby's mittens. Bilateral single transverse palmar creases may co-exist with other congenital abnormalities. Minor degrees of varus and valgus deformities of the feet are common. In these cases the foot can usually be slightly over-corrected by passive manipulation. A talipes equinovarus, where the foot cannot be manipulated to the normal position, requires immediate splinting.

The hips must be examined for congenital dislocation (Figure 25). The baby should lie supine on a flat surface, with the hips flexed at 90 degrees and the knees bent. With the upper part of the tibia resting in the hollow between the examiner's forefinger and thumb, the femur is gripped so that the middle finger is held over the greater trochanter and the thumb over the lesser trochanter. One hip is tested at a time.

First Movement

Adduct the hip, pressing laterally with the thumb. At the same time exert a downward pressure along the line of the thigh. The dislocatable hip will be felt to clunk over the posterior edge of the acetabulum.

Second Movement

Abduct the hip, pressing medially with the middle finger. A clunk is felt as the head of the femur returns to the acetabulum.

Parameters of Body Size

In addition to the measurement of body weight, the occipitofrontal head circumference and crown–heel length should be carefully recorded and plotted on a standard chart which relates these parameters to gestational age. This provides information concerning preceding intrauterine growth and also establishes a baseline against which subsequent growth may be compared.

Conclusion

Examination in the newborn period is the first in a series of 'checkups' an individual is likely to receive during a lifetime. The advent of hospital confinement and publicity about congenital malformations in the popular press and television has created an atmosphere which may lead a mother to assume that her baby is abnormal until proved otherwise. Perhaps the most important facet of the examination of the newborn is that in most cases it allows the mother to be reassured about the normality of her baby.

References

Harris, J. R. and Schick, B., *Am. J. Dis. Child.,* 1956, **92,** 27.
Pratt, A. G., *Arch. Derm.,* 1953, **67,** 302.
Solomon, L. M. and Esterly, N. B., *Neonatal Dermatology,* 1973, chapter 6, W. B. Saunders Company, London.
Taylor, W. B. and Bondurant, C. P., *Arch. Derm.,* 1957, **76,** 591.

Further Reading

Ritter, M. A., *Am. J. Dis. Child.,* 1973, **125,** 30.

4. The Low Birthweight Baby

ABOUT seven per cent of all babies weigh 2,500 g or less at birth and are defined as low birthweight (LBW). About two-thirds of these babies are pre-term (<37 weeks) and of the appropriate birthweight for gestational age. The remainder include babies with a wide range of maturity who are characterised by being underweight for their gestational age or 'small-for-dates' (SFD). These descriptions, which are now widely accepted, have led to a better understanding of the problems associated with LBW. However, the classification is an arbitrary one. It should be remembered that a baby may weigh more than 2,500 g and yet still be pre-term or SFD.

The classification and major hazards of the LBW baby are outlined in this chapter. A more detailed consideration of the individual diseases to which the LBW baby is prone appears in later chapters.

Assessment of Gestational Age

Every LBW baby should be examined in the newborn period so that the gestational age suspected by the date of the mother's last menstrual period, or as a result of antenatal investigations, may be confirmed or refuted. Postnatal assessment of gestational age is based on neurological findings and/or the appearance of certain external physical characteristics.

Neurological

As gestation advances in the normal fetus, flexor muscle tone increases and certain reflexes appear in chronological order. Estimation of gestational age may therefore be made by assessing the baby's posture in the supine and prone positions, resistance to passive movements and the presence of neonatal reflexes. Neurological assessment of gestational age is unreliable in ill babies. False results may be obtained if the examination is made within a few hours of birth or when the baby is sleepy.

Physical

Maturation of the fetus is associated with changes in the appearance of the skin, breast tissue, ears and genitalia which form a basis for the evaluation of gestational age.

No single neurological sign or physical feature provides an accurate assessment of gestational age. Several scoring systems have been devised whereby points are allocated for the presence of each individual characteristic. The total number of points scored is then related to gestational age. One such scoring system was described by Dubowitz et al. (1970) who combined ten neurological observations similar to those made by Amiel-Tison (1968) with 11 external physical characteristics described by Farr et al. (1966). (See Table 8 and Figures 26 and 27.) As with other methods of assessment the author's original instructions must be carefully followed. Proficiency and speed in performing the test improve with practice. Gestational age determined by this method is accurate to within ± two weeks.

A simpler method was described by Robinson (1966) who studied the time of appearance of a number of reflexes in babies of known gestational age between 25 and 42 weeks. Five reflexes appeared at predictable times irrespective of whether the baby was SFD or the appropriate weight for gestational age, and irrespective of whether the baby had been maturing inside or outside the uterus (Table 9). Although the test can be performed rapidly it is of limited value in distinguishing the gestational ages of babies more than 35 to 36 weeks.

Birthweight and Gestational Age: The Intrauterine Growth Chart

Many different charts or grids have been constructed which relate birthweight to gestational age. The distribution of birthweight at each gestational age may be expressed as the mean ± two standard deviations, or in terms of percentiles. For practical purposes the SFD baby may be defined as one whose birthweight is more than two standard deviations below the mean, or less than the tenth percentile for the gestational age (Figure 28). It will be apparent that a baby can only be described as being SFD in relation to the population which formed the subject matter for the intrauterine growth chart. The term SFD has more meaning if the baby observed is of the same population from which the intrauterine growth chart was derived. Fetal gender, maternal height, weight, parity, socio-economic status, nutritional status and geographical area of residence all influence the range of birthweight for a given gestational age.

Table 8. Assessment of gestational age. Physical criteria (adapted by Dubowitz *et al.* 1970; from Farr *et al.* 1966).

External Sign	Score 0	1	2	3	4
Oedema	Obvious oedema hands and feet: pitting over tibia	No obvious oedema hands and feet; pitting over tibia	No oedema		
Skin texture	Very thin, gelatinous	Thin and smooth	Smooth; medium thickness. Rash or superficial peeling	Slight thickening. Superficial cracking and peeling esp. hands & feet	Thick and parchment-like: superficial or deep cracking
Skin colour (infant not crying)	Dark red	Uniformly pink	Pale pink: variable over body	Pale. Only pink over ears, lips, palms or soles	
Skin opacity (trunk)	Numerous veins and venules clearly seen, especially over abdomen	Veins and tributaries seen	A few large vessels clearly seen over abdomen	A few large vessels seen indistinctly over abdomen	No blood vessels seen
Lanugo (over back)	No lanugo	Abundant; long and thick over whole back	Hair thinning especially over lower back	Small amount of lanugo and bald areas	At least half of back devoid of lanugo
Plantar creases	No skin creases	Faint red marks over anterior half of sole	Definite red marks over more than anterior half; indentations over less than anterior third	Indentations over more than anterior third	Definite deep indentations over more than anterior third
Nipple formation	Nipple barely visible; no areola	Nipple well defined; areola smooth and flat; diameter <0.75 cm	Areola stippled, edge not raised; diameter <0.75 cm	Areola stippled, edge raised; diameter >0.75 cm	
Breast size	No breast tissue palpable	Breast tissue on one or both sides <0.5 cm diameter	Breast tissue both sides; one or both 0.5–1.0 cm	Breast tissue both sides; one or both >1 cm	
Ear form	Pinna flat and shapeless, little or no incurving of edge	Incurving of part of edge of pinna	Partial incurving whole of upper pinna	Well-defined incurving whole of upper pinna	
Ear firmness	Pinna soft, easily folded, no recoil	Pinna soft, easily folded, slow recoil	Cartilage to edge of pinna, but soft in places, ready recoil	Pinna firm, cartilage to edge, instant recoil	
Genitalia (male)	Neither testis in scrotum	At least one testis high in scrotum	At least one testis right down		
Genitalia (female) (with hips half abducted)	Labia majora widely separated, labia minora protruding	Labia majora almost cover labia minora	Labia majora completely cover labia minora		

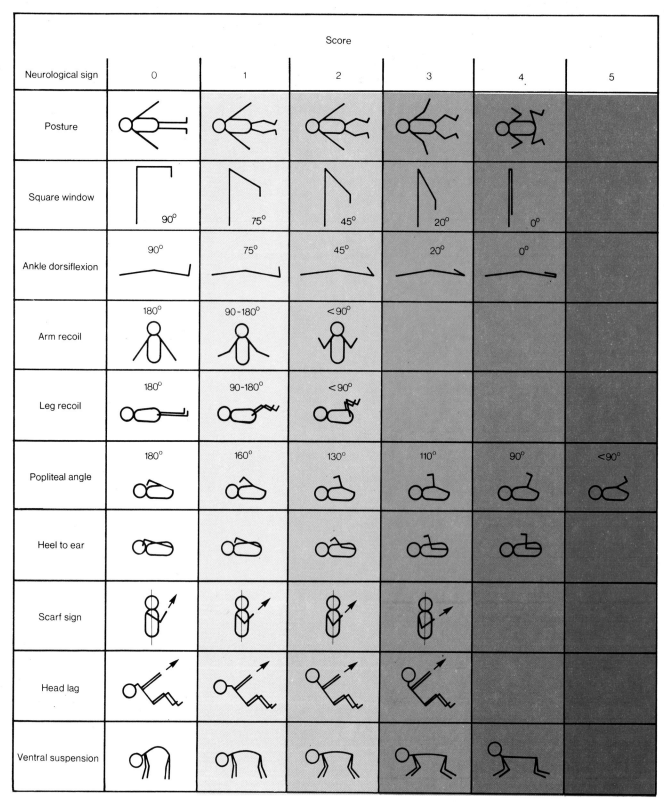

Figure 26. *Assessment of gestational age—neurological criteria (adapted by Dubowitz* et al. *1970 from Amiel-Tison 1968).*
Posture. *Observe with infant quiet and in supine position.*
Square window. *Flex hand on the forearm.* Ankle dorsiflexion. *Dorsiflex foot onto the anterior aspect of leg.*
Arm recoil. *Flex forearm for five seconds, then fully extend and release.*
Leg recoil. *Flex hip and knees for five seconds, then fully extend and release.*
Popliteal angle. *Hold thigh in the knee–chest position, then extend leg.*
Heel to ear. *Draw the foot near to head. Observe degree of extension of knee and distance between foot and head.*
Scarf sign. *Draw hand towards opposite shoulder.*
Grade position of elbow according to illustration.
Head lag. *Pull up slowly from supine position, grasping hands.*
Ventral suspension. *Suspend in prone position, holding under the chest.*

The Small-for-dates Baby

Aetiology

SFD babies form a heterogenous group of varied aetiology. There is interaction of many of the factors associated with fetal growth retardation and a single cause can rarely be ascertained (Table 10). The term 'placental insufficiency' is commonly used particularly where fetal growth retardation is associated with severe pre-eclamptic toxaemia, hypertension or recurrent antepartum bleeding. An expression best avoided, it wrongly implies that there often exists well-defined placental pathology which is the direct cause of poor fetal growth. In fact gross macroscopical lesions are only rarely detected in the placentae of SFD babies and 'gritty' or 'infarcted' placentae are sometimes seen in association with apparently normal babies.

The significance of the microscopic findings which have been reported inconstantly in the placentae of malnourished fetuses is debatable. Although the placentae of SFD babies are small, the ratio of placental/fetal bodyweight is normal (Scott and Usher 1966; Younoszai and Haworth 1969). The association of congenital malformations with SFD babies is of practical importance. About ten per cent of liveborn SFD babies have some form of major congenital abnormality. The most commonly reported intrauterine infections in association with fetal growth retardation are caused by cytomegalovirus and the rubella virus. The evidence that other intrauterine infections cause fetal growth retardation is less certain. Maternal nutritional intake in the last trimester of

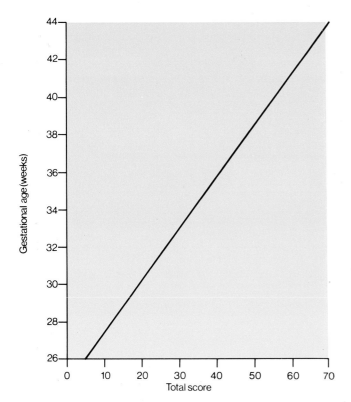

Figure 27. *Graph relating total score to gestational age.*

Figure 28. *Birthweight percentiles for gestational age (Butler and Alberman 1969).*
A. Full-term baby, appropriate weight for gestational age.
B. Full-term baby, small for dates.
C. Pre-term baby, appropriate weight for gestational age.
D. Pre-term baby, small for dates.

Table 9. Neonatal reflexes and gestational age (Robinson 1966).

Reflex	Gestational age (weeks) if reflex is	
	Present	Absent
Pupillary reaction to light	29 or more	< 31
Glabellar tap	32 or more	< 34
Head turning to diffuse light	32 or more	Doubtful
Traction	33 or more	< 36
Neck righting	34 or more	< 37

Glabellar tap. Blink of eyelids in response to a tap on glabella.
Head turning to diffuse light. Allow diffuse light to fall on one side of the face only. The head and eyes turn slowly towards the light.
Traction. Pull up by wrists from supine position. Observe for any one of: flexion of elbows, bracing of shoulders or raising of head.
Neck righting. Rotate head to one side. Observe for rotation of the trunk in the same direction.

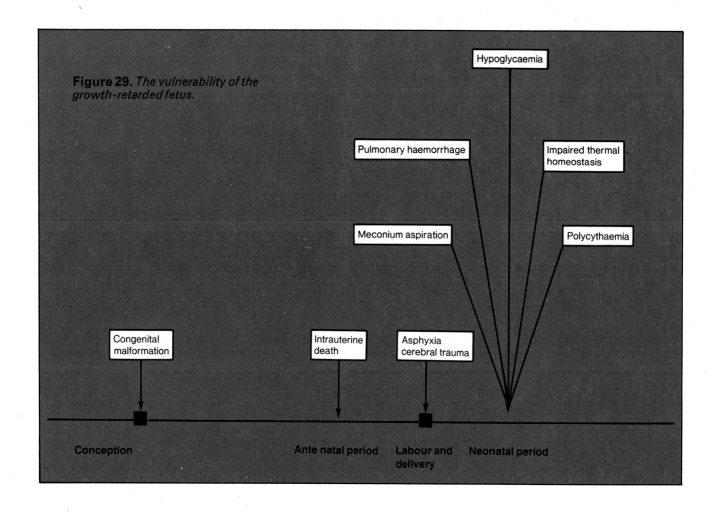

Figure 29. *The vulnerability of the growth-retarded fetus.*

Table 10. Some factors associated with fetal growth retardation.

Genetic.
Primiparity.
Maternal age under 20 years.
Deprived socio-economic class.
Maternal heroin addiction.
Maternal malnutrition.
Smoking.
Intrauterine infection (rubella ,cytomegalovirus).
Severe pre-eclamptic toxaemia or hypertension.
Recurrent antepartum bleeding.
Multiple pregnancy.
Congenital malformation.
Pregnancy at high altitude.

---

pregnancy influences fetal growth. There is strong evidence that the mean birthweight of a population is reduced by famine.

Body Composition

There is considerable variation in the degree to which different organs are affected in fetal growth retardation. The brain and heart are heavier in SFD babies compared with babies of a similar weight who are the appropriate weight for gestational age. By contrast the weights of the liver, lungs and thymus are lower (Gruenwald 1963).

Although there appears to be sparing of the brain in fetal growth retardation, weight is a crude reflection of organ growth. Using more sophisticated methods Dobbing (1974) showed that the human brain undergoes two separate growth spurts from 15 to 20 weeks and from 30 weeks to 18 months postnatal age. The developing brain is most vulnerable at times of rapid growth. The timing of fetal growth failure may be a critical factor in determining the outcome in terms of intellectual function.

Complications

The continuum of mortality and morbidity which forms the basis for an understanding of neonatal medicine is illustrated *par excellence* in the SFD baby who is especially vulnerable during the third trimester, during labour and delivery and in the neonatal period (Figure 29).

As gestation advances beyond 34 weeks the growth-retarded fetus has an increased risk of death *in utero* before the onset of labour. Excluding those fetuses with gross congenital malformations or intrauterine viral infections, the cause of death is unknown although it is commonly attributed to 'fetal asphyxia'. The risk of dying from asphyxia or cerebral trauma during labour and delivery is high before term, reaches a minimum at 40 weeks and rises again as gestation is prolonged beyond 40 weeks. The vulnerability of the SFD baby to asphyxia is partly related to the baby's low stores of liver and cardiac glycogen. The *neonatal mortality* becomes less as gestation advances to term. Some of the problems which face the SFD baby in the neonatal period are discussed below.

A common dilemma for the obstetrician and neonatal paediatrician is the management of the growth-retarded fetus. Allowing the fetus to remain inside a uterus which is not supporting growth exposes the fetus to an increasing risk of death *in utero* as gestation advances. On the other hand expediting delivery before term increases the risk of death during labour, delivery and the neonatal period.

Meconium Aspiration Syndrome

This is a form of respiratory distress which begins soon after birth. It is caused by the aspiration into the lungs of amniotic fluid contaminated with meconium. The occurrence of this condition in SFD babies is not surprising because gasping *in utero* and the passage of meconium into amniotic fluid are signs of fetal asphyxia to which the SFD fetus is prone.

Pulmonary Haemorrhage

The usual presentation is that of peripheral circulatory failure with the appearance of blood-stained fluid welling from the trachea. The condition is almost always fatal and most commonly occurs between two to four days of life. Although it may occur *de novo* it usually presents in a baby who has already suffered other insults such as birth asphyxia, meconium aspiration syndrome, etc. Cole *et al.* (1973) have suggested that the pathogenesis is acute left heart failure resulting in haemorrhagic pulmonary oedema.

Hypoglycaemia

A blood glucose level below 20 mg per cent (1.11 mmol/l) is a practical definition of hypoglycaemia in the newborn. The feeding of SFD babies with full-strength milk should begin soon after birth to help prevent hypoglycaemia which is probably caused by reduced hepatic glycogen stores and impaired gluconeogenesis. Symptomatic hypoglycaemia is more common in males and may present at any time in the first few days of life. Asymptomatic hypoglycaemia is detected by screening all SFD babies for hypoglycaemia, every eight hours in the first

Table 11. The vulnerability of the pre-term baby.

Idiopathic respiratory distress syndrome.
Apnoeic attacks.
Jaundice.
Impaired thermal homeostasis.
Feeding problems.
Functional intestinal obstruction.
Necrotising enterocolitis.
Infection.
Intraventricular or subarachnoid haemorrhage.

72 hours of life, with the 'Dextrostix' test (Ames Ltd).

Polycythaemia

This may be defined as a venous packed cell volume greater than 70 per cent. The susceptibility of SFD babies to polycythaemia is not fully understood. Symptoms and signs related to increased blood viscosity may occur, such as respiratory distress, cardiac failure, and convulsions. Jaundice is common because the large amount of bilirubin produced from the red-cell pool exceeds the capacity of the liver for conjugation.

Impaired Thermal Homeostasis

A large surface area relative to body weight and a reduced amount of subcutaneous fat render the SFD baby vulnerable to heat loss. Brown fat stores are reduced leading to impairment of non-shivering thermogenesis. The thermo-neutral environment suggested for babies of an appropriate weight for gestational age probably does not apply to SFD babies. It has been suggested by Sweet (1973) that the SFD baby is preferably nursed in an incubator adjusted to maintain the abdominal skin temperature between 36.0 °C and 36.5 °C.

The Pre-term Baby

Although numerous factors have been shown to be associated with the occurrence of premature delivery the cause, in most cases, is unknown. Those factors responsible for the normal onset of parturition in man are imperfectly understood. Cervical incompetence and other maternal complications of pregnancy are only associated with a small proportion of premature births.

Compared with the SFD baby, the pre-term baby is less at risk during labour and delivery, but is especially vulnerable during the neonatal period. The difficulties are those of adaptation to extra-uterine life in the face of immaturity of different organ systems. Some of the more common problems are briefly outlined in Table 11.

Idiopathic Respiratory Distress Syndrome (IRDS)

Lack of a normal surface active alveolar lining is the major aetiological factor in IRDS which is the most common cause of neonatal mortality in pre-term babies. Signs of respiratory distress are present at birth or develop within one or two hours. The overall incidence in pre-term babies is about ten per cent and the highest incidence occurs in pre-term babies weighing between 1,000 g and 1,500 g.

Impaired Thermal Homeostasis

The pre-term baby shares with the SFD baby problems of thermal homeostasis. Instead of enjoying maternal homeothermy he has to call upon his reserves of brown fat which are small in relation to body weight compared with his full-term counterpart. There are important practical reasons for ensuring that the pre-term baby is nursed within the thermo-neutral range. The neonatal mortality is higher, and growth rate in terms of body weight and length is smaller under conditions of cold stress.

Feeding

The pre-term baby cannot suck satisfactorily, has impaired swallowing, imperfect development of those reflex mechanisms which protect the air passages from liquids intended for the stomach, and has a small stomach volume. With these handicaps he strives to mimic intra-uterine growth with a food (milk) which has a quite different nutrient quality compared with the 'food' he would have been receiving across the placenta. In spite of this, total intravenous nutrition, which has many hazards, has not shown to be superior to milk feeding in premature babies. Feeding of small volumes of milk by the nasogastric route is favoured in most neonatal units.

Jaundice

'Physiological' jaundice is characterised by its occurrence after the first 36 hours of life, rising to a peak of up to 12 mg per cent by the fourth or fifth day and gradually falling to < 1.5 mg per cent by the tenth day.[1] The reason usually given for the relatively high incidence of this type of jaundice in pre-term babies is that there is a reduced amount of glucuronyl transferase, the liver enzyme responsible for bilirubin conjugation. This is undoubtedly an oversimplification because several factors contribute to the aetiology of 'physiological' jaundice. However, of much greater significance is the fact that pre-term babies are liable to develop kernicterus at lower levels of serum bilirubin than full-term babies. This influences the management of the jaundice.

Apnoeic Attacks

Recurrent cessation of breathing sometimes associated with cyanosis and bradycardia may begin in the first few days of life or the onset may be delayed until the second week. A cause can rarely be found. While in many cases simple external stimulation will restart breathing, death in association with recurrent apnoea is common in pre-term babies. The necropsy demonstration of an intra-ventricular or subarachnoid haemorrhage is often made, but its presence is not necessarily causal.

Intracranial Haemorrhage

Intraventricular and subarachnoid haemorrhages are often associated with previous episodes of hypoxia. Therefore it is not surprising that such haemorrhages are a frequent necropsy finding in pre-term babies who have died with IRDS or recurrent apnoeic attacks. The clinical presentation is that of shock with neurological signs including convulsions, squinting and 'sun-setting' appearance of the eyes. There is often a fall in body temperature, blood pH, and arterial oxygen tension. The condition is uniformly fatal in babies who develop these signs.

Infection

Impaired humoral and cellular defence mechanisms render the pre-term baby vulnerable to infection. Life-threatening conditions which may present with ill-defined symptoms and signs include septicaemia and meningitis. The routine use of prophylactic antibiotics in pre-term babies is not desirable. Vigilance by nursing and medical staff is required so that early signs or symptoms of infection, such as any change in behaviour of the baby, may be recognised.

The Outcome in Low Birthweight Babies

Several centres throughout the world have noted an increased neonatal survival rate, particularly among very LBW babies (< 1500 g), with the institution of modern methods of perinatal care. Survival rates ranging from 50 to 75 per cent have been reported, although when interpreting these figures it is important to consider the author's concepts of viability in those extremely small babies who fulfil the definition of being live-born.

The neurological sequelae and later intelligence of LBW babies have been expertly reviewed by Davies and Stewart (1975). Diverse factors contribute to the long-term outcome. In individual babies such factors include the following:

1. Genetic endowment.

2. The nature of perinatal and neonatal complications.

3. The standard of care received.

4. The degree of mother/baby contact in the neonatal unit.

5. Environmental factors operating after discharge from hospital.

The most common form of cerebral palsy in LBW babies was spastic diplegia. The incidence was shown to be inversely correlated with gestational age suggesting that prematurity was an important aetiological factor. During the past 15 years there has been a striking reduction in the incidence of spastic diplegia among very low LBW babies. Individual centres now report an incidence below four per cent (Fitzhardinge and Steven 1972; Stewart and Reynolds 1974), whereas in earlier surveys the incidence was ten to 30 per cent. The incidence of other forms of cerebral palsy, such as hemiplegia and quadriplegia, is also lower now compared with earlier reports.

However, in the absence of overt cerebral palsy careful follow-up of LBW babies sometimes reveals minor impairment of function or 'clumsiness' (*Lancet* 1973). The recognition of the role of oxygen toxicity in the aetiology of retrolental fibroplasia has led to a reduction in the incidence of serious visual handicap in LBW babies from around ten to 20 per cent to one to two per cent. The incidence of sensorineural hearing loss has fallen from around ten per cent to one to two per cent in the

---

[1]Throughout the book bilirubin levels are expressed in mg per cent. These levels may be converted to SI units (μmol/l) by multiplying by 17.1. To convert bilirubin in μmol/l to mg per cent, multiply the value by 0.06.

past 20 years. This may be partly caused by improved management of hyperbilirubinaemia. Data concerning the subsequent intelligence quotient (IQ) of LBW babies have to be interpreted with caution, because the IQ of the parents and the degree of intellectual stimulation provided at home are potent factors which influence the results. The nature of the IQ test should also be considered because a 'normal' IQ result may mask certain areas of handicap. Nevertheless, there is still good evidence that there has been an improvement in the mean IQ of LBW babies during the last 15 years (Davies and Stewart 1975).

Conclusions

The reduction in neonatal mortality and the improved long-term prognosis in LBW babies are attributable in part to improved standards of perinatal and neonatal care. Facilities for the intensive care of LBW babies no longer have to be justified. An understanding of the physiology of growth and adaptation from conception, through birth, to the neonatal period forms the basis of good neonatal care.

References

Amiel-Tison, C., *Arch. Dis. Childh.,* 1968, **43**, 89.

Butler, N. R. and Alberman, E. D., *Perinatal Problems,* E. & S. Livingstone, Edinburgh 1969.

Cole, V., Normand, I. and Reynolds, E., *Pediatrics,* 1973, **51**, 175.

Davies, P. A. and Stewart, A. L., *Br. Med. Bull.,* 1975, **31**, 85.

Dobbing, J., In *Scientific Foundations of Paediatrics* (p. 565), (Ed. Davis, J. A. and Dobbing, J.), William Heinemann Ltd., London, 1974.

Dubowitz, L., Dubowitz,V. and Goldberg, C., *J. Pediat.,* 1970, **77**, 1.

Farr, V., Mitchell, R. and Neligan, G., *Devlop. Med. Child Neurol.,* 1966, **8**, 507.

Fitzhardinge, P. M. and Steven, E. M., *Pediatrics,* 1972, **50**, 50.

Gruenwald, P., *Biol. Neonat.,* 1963, **5**, 215.

Lancet, 1973, **2**, 487.

Robinson, R. J., *Arch. Dis. Childh.,* 1966, **41**, 437.

Scott, K. E. and Usher, R., *Am. J. Obstet. Gynecol.,* 1966, **94**, 951.

Stewart, A. L. and Reynolds, E. O. R., *Pediatrics,* 1974, **54**, 724.

Sweet, A. Y., In *Care of the High Risk Neonate* (p. 49), (Ed. Klaus, M. H. and Fanaroff, A. A.), W. B. Saunders, Philadelphia, 1973.

Younoszai, M. K. and Haworth, J. C., *Am. J. Obstet. Gynecol.,* 1969, **103**, 265.

Further Reading

Lubchenco, L. O., Searls, D. T. and Brazie, J. V., *J. Pediatr.,* 1972, **81**, 814.

5. Nutrition

THE nutritional consequences of separation of the baby from the maternal blood supply at birth are no less important than the respiratory implications. The new-born baby has an innate capacity to breathe, but is wholly dependent on his care-giver for adequate nutrition.

The baby, unlike the adult, has to contend with growth, and so an understanding of nutrition is of special relevance in the neonatal period.

Growth

Fetal growth accelerates during the last six months of gestation, and towards the end weight gain is 35 g per day. This rate falls to 30 g per day by two months postnatal age and later declines throughout infancy (Figure 30). In spite of these fluctuations in growth rate, a normal baby gains about the same amount of weight during the first 20 weeks after birth as during the last 20 weeks before birth.

An alternative way of expressing growth is weight gain per day as a percentage of bodyweight. There is a six per cent increase in fetal weight per day at the end of the first trimester. Thereafter, growth expressed as a percentage increase in body weight per day falls progressively until six months postnatal age, except for the period between 26 and 32 weeks of intrauterine life when there is a brief increase (Figure 30).

The normal baby loses weight during the first few days after birth and this largely represents loss of body water. Such losses normally do not exceed ten per cent of the birthweight and by the tenth day the normal baby does not weigh less than his birthweight.

Fetal Nutrition

The function of the placenta as an organ of fetal growth is imperfectly understood. It is certain that the fetus does not receive all nutrients via the placenta simply as an ultrafiltrate of maternal plasma. Several different mechanisms are responsible for the placental transfer of nutrients, and the placenta plays a role in the synthesis of certain materials such as proteins, nucleic acids, and enzymes.

Glucose is continuously being transferred across the placenta and is the major source of energy for the fetus. Glycogen is synthesised and stored in the liver and heart.

There is rapid use of stored glycogen from the moment of birth, when the maternal supply of glucose is cut off and when gluconeogenesis has not yet become established.

White fat is laid down in increasing amounts during the latter half of pregnancy and the fetus is able to synthesise fatty acids. It is not known whether a significant transfer of fatty acids across the placenta occurs.

The concentration of amino acids in fetal blood is greater than that in maternal blood. An active placental transport mechanism is thought to be responsible, different amino acids being taken up with varying degrees of avidity by the fetus.

Neonatal Nutrition
Energy

The total caloric value of mature human milk is about 67 cal per 100 ml. Most full-cream cow's milk preparations used for feeding normal babies have a similar energy value to human milk, but certain half-cream milks have a smaller energy value (55 cal per 100 ml).

Figure 30. *Percentage daily weight gain (black), and absolute daily weight gain (g) (red) during the last six months of fetal life and the first six months after birth (adapted from Usher and McClean 1974).*

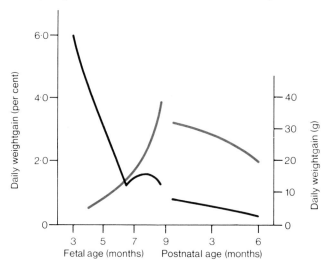

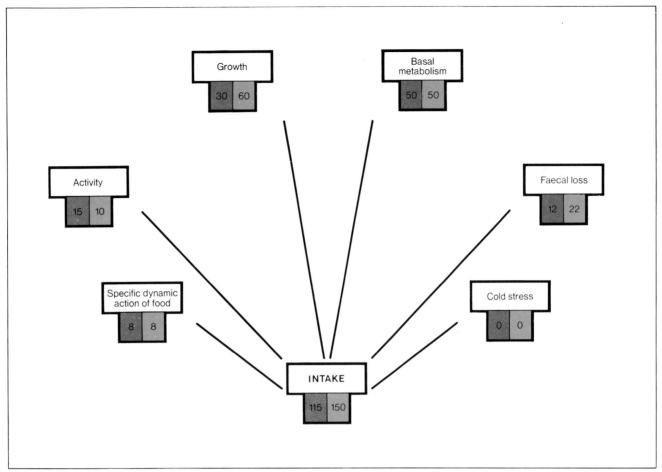

Figure 31. *Approximate distribution of energy intake (cal/kg/day) in the neonatal period of a full-term baby (3 kg) blue boxes, and premature baby (1 kg) red boxes, nursed within the thermoneutral range and thereby not subjected to cold stress.*

The caloric intake of healthy neonates varies considerably. There is a sharp increase in caloric intake during the first week of life in babies fed *ad libitum*, and thereafter intake is about 110 to 120 cal/kg/day, equivalent to a volume of milk of 160 to 180 ml/kg/day. The normal baby can to some extent regulate the volume of milk taken according to its caloric concentration. Foman *et al.* (1971) showed that babies fed with dilute milk (53 cal per 100 ml) ingested a greater volume of milk (ml/kg/day) compared with babies fed milk of a conventional caloric value (67 cal per 100 ml).

The various compartments of energy expenditure for a full-term and premature neonate are shown in Figure 31. The energy expenditure for growth in the full-term neonate approaches 30 per cent of the total caloric intake because so much protein and fat is being laid down.

The very premature baby is at a disadvantage in terms of caloric balance in a number of ways. The caloric cost of growth is very high (about 40 per cent of the total caloric intake) because of the rapid rate of growth which ought to be achieved after birth and which would have been achieved had the baby remained *in utero*. The faecal loss of calories in the form of fat is greater compared with normal babies. The premature baby is more likely to be subject to cold stress. Valuable calories will be diverted from growth towards the maintenance of a normal body temperature unless the baby is carefully nursed within the thermoneutral range. In addition, Mestyán *et al.* (1968) observed considerable increase in physical activity in premature babies nursed in an environment which was too cold, and this also represents caloric wastage. The caloric requirement for a premature neonate is at least 150 cal/kg/day, even when the baby is nursed in a suitable thermal environment.

Protein

The protein requirement for a normal baby in the first six weeks of life is 2 g/kg/day, and 70 per cent of this requirement is used for growth. A baby receiving 180 ml/kg/day of human milk would have a protein intake of about 2 g/kg/day. Unmodified cow's milk contains three times as much protein (3.3 g per 100 ml) as human milk (1.2 g per 100 ml), and the same baby fed with cow's milk would have a protein intake of about 6 g/kg/day. There is no evidence that such a large protein intake *per se* causes superior growth, but it is associated with abnormally high blood-urea levels (Davies and Saunders 1973). Modified cow's-milk preparations are available with protein concentrations of 1.5 to 2.7 g per 100 ml.

Human milk has a high ratio of whey protein (60 per cent) to casein (40 per cent) compared with cow's milk (whey 20 per cent, casein 80 per cent). The relatively large concentration of casein in cow's milk may lead to the formation of insoluble curds in the stomach. This has been implicated as a cause of intestinal obstruction in the newborn (Cook and Rickham 1969). The whey: casein protein ratio approximates to that of human milk in certain 'humanised' milk preparations in which de-mineralised whey is added to non-fat cow's milk. The amino acid pattern of human and cow's milk differs considerably, but there is nothing to suggest that either milk offers specific advantages over the other in terms of growth.

The protein requirement for optimal growth in premature babies is unknown but is likely to be about 3 to 4 g/kg/day (Foman 1974). Protein intakes in excess of 4 g/kg/day are best avoided. Superior weight gain in association with a very high protein intake is probably largely caused by water retention as a result of an increased solute load. Abnormally high levels of certain plasma amino acids have been detected in premature babies fed with high-protein diets (Valman *et al.* 1971).

Fat

The fat of milk is mainly in the form of triglyceride (Figure 32). The fatty acid radical of the triglyceride may be of long, medium or short chain type depending on the number of carbon atoms forming the chain. The fatty acids are further classified into those that are saturated and have no 'double-bond' links between the carbon atoms, and those that are unsaturated and have a variable number of 'double-bond' links between carbon atoms. Palmitic acid (long chain, saturated) and oleic acid (long chain, unsaturated) comprise 60 per cent of the total fatty acids in human and cow's milk.

Although newborn babies have a relatively low pancreatic lipase activity and small amounts of bile salts in their intestine, they are able to absorb 90 per cent of their intake of human milk fat. In contrast only 60 to 65 per cent of their intake of cow's milk fat is absorbed. Some reasons for this are summarised in Table 12. Human milk contains a greater percentage of unsaturated fatty acids which are hydrolysed more readily by pancreatic lipase. Palmitic acid, which is quantitatively the most important saturated fatty acid, is better absorbed not as a free fatty acid but attached to glycerol in the '2' position as a monoglyceride. In human milk 75 per cent of palmitic acid is in the '2' position, whereas in cow's milk only 40 per cent of palmitic acid is in the '2' position. In some proprietary milk preparations, milk fat is replaced with a blend of other fats and oils so that the mixture of fatty

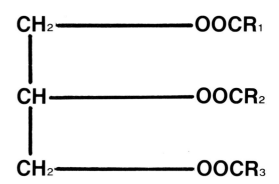

Figure 32. *Structure of triglyceride. R_1, R_2, R_3, represent fatty acids which may be of long, medium or short chain length and which may be saturated or unsaturated.*

acids obtained approximates more closely to that of human milk.

It would appear that fat absorption is equally impaired in premature and small-for-date babies (Barltrop and Oppé 1973). This is an important cause of caloric wastage in low birthweight babies.

Carbohydrate

Carbohydrate is present in milk in the form of lactose and there is a greater concentration in human milk (7 g per 100 ml) compared with cow's milk (4.8 g per 100 ml). At the brush border of the small intestine lactose is split by lactase into glucose and galactose, which are then absorbed by an active transport mechanism. A relative deficiency of intestinal lactase in the first few weeks of life may explain the rather frequent loose stools of normal breast-fed babies in the newborn period. Sugar in the form of sucrose has to be added to certain unmodified cow's-milk preparations. Intestinal sucrase is present from birth and sucrose is readily absorbed, provided excess amounts are not added to the milk.

Calcium and Phosphorus

About 28 mg per kg body weight of calcium is laid down daily during the first few months of life. The calcium content of human milk is 33 mg per 100 ml and most proprietary milk preparations contain two or three times this amount. Once feeding has become established the intake of calcium would exceed 28 mg/kg/day. The problem is that calcium is poorly absorbed. The calcium retention is only just equal to the estimated requirements

Table 12. Chemical characteristics and absorption of human and cow's milk fat.

	Fat absorption (per cent)	Unsaturated fatty acids (per cent of total fat)	Palmitic acid in '2' position (per cent of total palmitic acid)
Mature human milk	90	48	75
Cow's milk	60 to 65	35	40

for growth in babies fed with human milk. The calcium retention in babies fed with cow's milk preparations varies considerably with the type of preparation used and is strongly influenced by the amount of fat in the milk. Faecal excretion of fat and calcium is positively correlated. There is some evidence that calcification of the long bones of babies during early infancy does not keep pace with new matrix formation (Dickerson 1962).

About 20 mg/kg body weight of phosphorus is laid down daily in the first few months of life. The phosphorus content of human milk is 15 mg per 100 ml and many proprietary milks contain three to five times this amount. Babies fed with human milk retain sufficient phosphate for growth, but babies fed with certain cow's milk preparations retain far more phosphate than is required. The kidneys of the newborn baby have difficulty in excreting a large phosphate load, and there occurs a rise in the serum phosphate level and a reciprocal fall in the serum calcium level. This is probably the major aetiological factor in hypocalcaemic tetany of the newborn, which presents towards the end of the first week of life and which does not occur in wholly breast-fed babies.

Sodium

The sodium content of human milk is 15 mg per 100 ml whereas the sodium content of cow's milk is 58 mg per 100 ml. The clinical relevance of sodium in nutrition is the danger of an excess sodium intake in babies fed with cow's milk preparations. This is particularly liable to occur when the feeds are incorrectly reconstituted so that the concentration is too high. Hypernatraemia may result, particularly if a baby has a concurrent infection causing abnormal loss of water. Demineralised milk preparations are available which have a sodium concentration more in keeping with that of human milk.

Iron

The total iron content of the full-term baby at birth is about 300 mg. Most of the iron is in the circulating red-cell mass and only 20 mg represents tissue stores.

During the first six to eight weeks of life there is a reduction in the red-cell mass and iron released from the circulation is stored. Erythropoiesis becomes active at about eight to 12 weeks and at this time the iron stores are used. Human and cow's milk contain very little iron (0.1 to 0.15 mg per 100 ml) and a baby is largely dependent on stored iron for normal erythropoiesis. Fortunately iron stores in a full-term baby are usually sufficient to prevent the occurrence of iron-deficiency anaemia.

The premature baby after birth has a smaller red-cell mass and tissue stores of iron compared with the full-term baby. Consequently the total amount of iron released from the circulating red-cell mass in the first six to eight weeks is smaller. When erythropoiesis is resumed at eight to 12 weeks the iron stores are exhausted. A hypochromic iron-deficiency anaemia may develop from the age of 16 weeks unless supplemental iron is given.

Iron given shortly after birth in the form of a ferrous sulphate supplemented milk preparation to achieve an intake of 2.5 mg/kg/day builds up the premature baby's iron stores and prevents iron-deficiency anaemia (Dollman 1974). This intake is difficult to achieve even with available milk preparations which contain relatively large iron supplements (1.2 mg per 100 ml). The alternative is to give medicinal iron (2.5 mg/kg/day). Ferrous amino aceto sulphate has been beneficial in preventing the development of iron-deficiency anaemia of prematurity.

There is a relationship between iron and vitamin E which has implications for the premature baby in the first two months of life. Iron is a co-factor that catalyses the oxidative breakdown of the lipid membrane of the red cell. In the face of a relative deficiency of vitamin E which normally protects the red-cell membrane from breakdown, the giving of iron prophylactically in the first two months may predispose the baby to a haemolytic anaemia. It may be prudent to delay giving iron to premature babies until after eight weeks.

Vitamins

The recommended doses of vitamins which are commonly given to babies are shown in Table 13.

Vitamin K

Vitamin K has special implications during the first few days of life when a mild deficiency is liable to occur, particularly in babies who are fed with human milk. The clinical manifestation of the deficiency, haemorrhagic disease of the newborn, occurs in one in 400 babies. Every baby should receive a single parenteral dose (0.5 to 1.0 mg) of vitamin K_1 (phytylmenaquinone) soon after birth.

Vitamin A

A wide range of recommended daily intake is suggested by different authorities (500 to 1,500 IU). The lower end of the range more than suffices to prevent the occurrence of clinical manifestations of vitamin A deficiency (Foman 1974). Human and cow's milk are relatively rich sources of vitamin A, and a daily intake of 400 to 500 ml of either milk would provide 500 IU of vitamin A. Modified dried milk and 'ready to feed' formulae are fortified with vitamin A. In practice there would seem to be little need to provide medicinal vitamin A for babies of normal birthweight. The daily intake of 20,000 IU of vitamin A for one to two months is likely to be toxic (Foman 1974).

Vitamin C

The recommended daily intake is 15 to 20 mg. Human milk is normally a rich source of vitamin C and a daily intake of 400 to 500 ml would supply the recommended intake. Unmodified cow's-milk is a poor source of vitamin C. Dried milk and 'ready to feed' formulae are fortified with vitamin C, but they have a wide range of final vitamin C concentration. The recommended intake would only just be fulfilled with a daily intake of 500 ml using some preparations, and medicinal supplementation (20 mg daily) is desirable and safe.

Table 13. Recommended[1] daily intake of vitamins and vitamin content of milk.

	Recommended intake (daily)	Approximate content in 500 ml mature human milk	Approximate content in 500 ml powdered cow's milk supplemented with vitamins A, C and D.
Vitamin A (IU)	500 to 1,500	500 to 1,000	1,250 to 1,750
Vitamin C (mg)	15 to 20	20	15 to 25
Vitamin D (IU)	400	4.0	180 to 200
Folic acid (µg)	50	25	10
Vitamin E (IU)[2]	5 to 25	2.5	1.5

The recommended intakes of folic acid and vitamin E refer to premature babies. Every baby should receive a single parenteral dose (0.5 to 1.0 mg) of vitamin K_1 soon after birth.
[1] Foman (1974).
[2] Wide range of recommendations from different authorities.

Vitamin D

There is no dietary requirement for vitamin D with adequate exposure to sunlight. Sunlight alone is not sufficient to produce enough vitamin D by skin irradiation to prevent rickets in the UK. The recommended daily intake is 400 IU. Human and cow's milks are relatively poor sources of vitamin D, and even though commercially available cow's-milk preparations are fortified with the vitamin (36 to 44 IU per 100 ml), a baby would have to ingest 1,000 ml of milk daily to meet the recommended intake. Medicinal supplementation is necessary to bring the daily intake up to 400 IU. Intakes in excess of 1,000 IU daily should be avoided.

There is no evidence that full-term babies suffer harm if medicinal supplements of vitamins C and D are begun at one month rather than soon after birth. This arrangement ensures that the mother is unhampered by medicinal concerns during the very important period when she is coming to terms with her baby with regard to feeding.

The premature baby is handicapped by the fact that even when a milk is fortified with vitamins, the daily volume of milk ingested is likely to be small. In addition to vitamin K administration soon after birth, medicinal supplements of vitamins A, C and D should be given from the first few days of life. Vitamin requirements for the premature baby are largely unknown, and until there is evidence to the contrary the dose should be the same as for full-term babies. Folic acid and vitamin E have special implications for premature babies.

Folic Acid

Premature babies often have a low serum concentration of folic acid from two to six weeks after birth. When erythropoiesis resumes at six to eight weeks there is a demand for folic acid. A megaloblastic anaemia may occur if this demand is not met. A daily dose of 50 µg folic acid from birth until the introduction of solids prevents the occurrence of subnormal serum folic acid levels.

Vitamin E

One metabolic role of vitamin E is the protection of cell membranes against oxidative breakdown of lipids. The serum vitamin E level is often subnormal in very premature babies during the first two or three months of life, and body stores of the vitamin are low. Clinical manifestations of vitamin E deficiency, including haemolytic anaemia, oedema and a watery nasal discharge, may occur at this time. The desirable vitamin E intake is greater in babies receiving modified cow's milk preparations containing relatively large amounts of polyunsaturated fats. It would seem prudent to give premature babies 5 to 25 IU of a water-soluble preparation of vitamin E (α tocopherol acetate) during their first three months of life.

Conclusion

Nutrition has special implications for the developing organism. Normal weight gain is but a small reflection of the adequacy of nutrition. The influence of diet in the newborn period on brain development, intellectual achievement and the later development of certain diseases is a problem which remains largely unsolved.

References

Barltrop, D. and Oppé, T. E., *Arch. Dis. Child.*, 1973, **48**, 496.

Cook, R. C. M. and Rickham, P. P., *J. Pediat. Surg.*, 1969, **4**, 599.

Davies, D. P. and Saunders, P., *Arch. Dis. Child.*, 1973, **48**, 563.

Dickerson, J. W. T., *Biochem. J.*, 1962, **82**, 56.

Dollman, P. R., *J. Pediat.*, 1974, **85**, 742.

Foman, S. J., *Infant Nutrition*, W. B. Saunders Co., Philadelphia and London, 1974.

Foman, S. J., Thomas, L. N., Filer, L. J., Jr., Ziegler, E. E. and Leonard, M. T., *Acta Paediat.*, 1971, supplement 223.

Mestyán, J., Járai, I. and Fekete, M., *Pediat. Res.*, 1968, **2**, 161.

Usher, R. H. and McLean, F. H., *Scientific Foundations of Paediatrics*, (Ed. Davis, J. A. and Dobbing, J.), William Heinemann Medical Books Ltd., 1974.

Valman, H. B., Brown, R. J. K., Palmer, T., Oberholzer, V. G. and Levin, B., *Brit. Med. J.*, 1971, **4**, 789.

6. Infection

Mortality and morbidity from neonatal infection are considerably less now compared with the beginning of the century. This is largely because of improved standards of hygiene and the introduction of antibiotics. The present-day implications with respect to neonatal infection are different from those of 50 years ago when pneumonia and epidemic gastroenteritis were particularly common. There is now considerable awareness of:

1. The impact of infection acquired before birth and its role in premature delivery, stillbirth and fetal damage.

2. The importance of Gram-negative bacteria as a cause of neonatal infection.

3. The subtle symptomatology of the neonate who often reacts in a similar way to widely different infective agents regardless of the site of infection.

4. The special vulnerability of the premature baby to infection. Improved standards of supportive care have led to a greater number of very premature babies surviving beyond the first few days of life and becoming exposed to the risks of infection throughout the neonatal period.

5. The use of invasive practical techniques such as mechanical ventilation, umbilical vessel catheterisation, etc., which carry the risk of introducing infection.

Routes of Infection

Infection may be acquired in the uterus, during passage through the birth canal, or after birth. Special predilection of certain organisms for a particular route of attack is recognised. Transplacental passage of organisms from the maternal blood stream is the most important route of fetal infection. The fetus, by virtue of existence within a closed sterile sac, is to some extent protected against ascending colonisation from the birth canal and from contiguous spread of infection from surrounding structures such as the peritoneal cavity. However, the membranes, even when intact, are not a completely efficient barrier against infection. Once the membranes have ruptured the risk of fetal infection is positively correlated with the membrane rupture/delivery interval. During passage through the birth canal the fetus is exposed to the vaginal and perineal organisms of the mother. After birth the baby is at the mercy of his environment which includes the hands of his attendants and any apparatus that he might come into contact with. As far as the fetus and newborn are concerned any organism is potentially pathogenic. The outcome following the acquisition of an organism is heavily influenced by the defence mechanism of the host.

Defence Against Infection

Several defence mechanisms may be called into action to protect the neonate against infection (Figure 33).

Humoral Bactericidal System

This is a cell-free system involving a susceptible organism, antibody and complement.

Phagocytic System (Humoral Mediated)

The circulating polymorphonuclear leukocyte acts in conjunction with humoral factors (opsonin) which prepare the organism for phagocytosis. Specific antibody to the organism and certain components of complement act as opsonin in the reaction which entails antigen (organism)–antibody reaction, complement fixation, leukotaxis, ingestion and killing of the organism. Lysozymes

Figure 33. *Immunological mechanisms which defend the neonate against infection.*

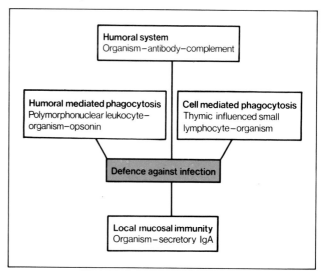

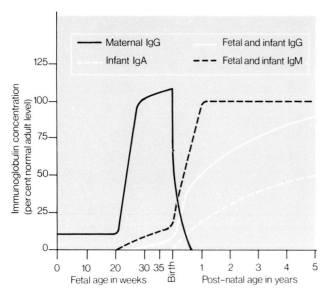

Figure 34. *The development of immunoglobulins in fetal and postnatal life.*

within the leukocyte contain many enzymes which play a role in the killing and degradation of the organism.

Phagocytic System (Cell Mediated)

The essential elements in cellular immunity are the immuno-competent small lymphocytes which are derived from marrow stem cells and gain their immuno-competence through the influence of thymic tissue. The system is mainly responsible for defence against organisms which are capable of surviving and multiplying within tissues, for example viruses, fungi, mycobacteria.

Local Mucosal Immunity

Secretory IgA is two molecules of ordinary IgA connected by a 'secretory piece' which is produced in epithelial cells. The molecule, which is not digested by proteolytic enzymes, has a particular role in protecting against respiratory and gastrointestinal infection by the neutralisation of viruses and the lysis of certain bacteria.

Effectiveness of Neonatal Defence Mechanisms

The capacity of the neonate to deal appropriately with organisms is limited. A gene locus for immunoglobulin synthesis on the X chromosome accounts in part for the greater susceptibility of the male neonate to infection. The development of immunoglobulins in fetal and postnatal life is shown in Figure 34. IgG is the only class of immunoglobulin which is transmitted across the placenta from the mother and offers the neonate some protection against those organisms which have IgG as their primary antibody, for example poliovirus, *Streptococcus* and *Haemophilus influenzae*. The fetus synthesises IgG in small amounts from the 20th week of gestation onwards. However, after birth the amounts synthesised do not compensate for the rapid disappearance of maternally derived IgG, so that serum IgG levels decline in the postnatal period to a nadir at three to five months. IgM anti-

bodies are not transported across the placenta from the mother but are synthesised by the fetus in small amounts from the 20th week of gestation onwards. The low serum concentration of IgM in the newborn compared with the adult is probably responsible for susceptibility to infection with Gram-negative bacteria which have IgM as their primary antibody. There is a rapid increase in IgM synthesis after birth, although the increase is slower in premature babies. IgA is neither transmitted across the placenta nor synthesised by the fetus. It is usually detected in small amounts in the serum by the second week of life, but appears in secretions soon after birth.

Total serum complement concentration at birth is less than in adults although certain components of complement have been detected in fetal sera as early as 12 to 15 weeks gestation. The humoral-mediated phagocytic system in respect of opsonification, leukotaxis and intracellular killing, is impaired in the newborn, particularly in those born prematurely. The occurrence of viraemia with a good circulating antibody response in the neonate suggests that the cell-mediated phagocytic system is deficient, although the precise nature of the deficiency is unclear.

Intrauterine Infection

A variety of organisms may be responsible for fetal infection (Table 14) and a wide spectrum of clinical events may result (Figure 35). The precise range of effects which may result from fetal infection with many individual organisms is unclear.

Non-Bacterial Infections

Of the many non-bacterial fetal infections which have been described, those due to cytomegalovirus, rubella virus and *Toxoplasma gondii* are of particular interest by virtue of their frequency and adverse effect on the host. The three organisms may produce a similar acute clinical picture in the neonatal period, consisting of anaemia, jaundice, thrombocytopenic purpura and hepatosplenomegaly. The combination of physical signs, which also occurs with bacterial septicaemia and severe rhesus haemolytic disease, should alert medical staff to the possibility of non-bacterial fetal infection.

Cytomegalovirus

Cytomegalovirus disease is one of the most common non-bacterial fetal infections. Approximately four to five per cent of women acquire primary cytomegalovirus infection during pregnancy and it is more prevalent in women who are socio-economically deprived. In the majority of cases the infection is asymptomatic. The risk of fetal infection is greater when the mother becomes infected in the first half of pregnancy. Abortion, stillbirth, premature delivery and fetal growth retardation are all associated with intrauterine cytomegalovirus infection, although the association may not always represent a cause and effect phenomenon.

The incidence of congenital cytomegalovirus infection in liveborn babies is 0.2 to 2.0 per cent. It is probable that

Table 14. Fetal infection—some causative organisms and routes of infection.

Infection acquired in ante-partum period:

Transplacental	*Ascending*
Cytomegalovirus	Candida albicans
Rubella virus	Herpes simplex
Poliovirus	Cytomegalovirus
Herpes simplex	Mycoplasma hominis
Hepatitis-associated antigen	Listeria monocytogenes
Toxoplasma gondii	Vibrio fetus
Treponema pallidum	Other vaginal and
Mycobacterium tuberculosis	perineal bacteria,
Other bacteria associated	including group B
with maternal septicaemia.	streptococcus.

Infection acquired during passage through birth canal:

Candida albicans
Herpes simplex
Cytomegalovirus
Mycoplasma hominis
Neisseria gonorrhoeae
TRIC agent
Pathogenic strains of Escherichia coli
Other vaginal and perineal bacteria

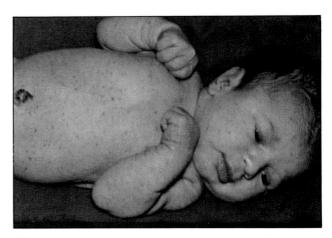

Figure 36. *Congenital cytomegalovirus infection. The virus was isolated from the urine of this neonate who has a widespread purpuric rash associated with thrombocytopenia.*

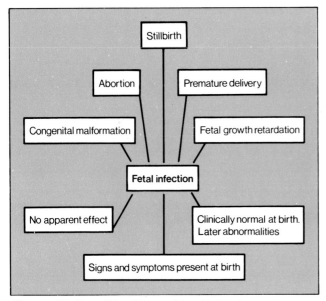

Figure 35. *Possible effects of fetal infection.*

only five to ten per cent of infected fetuses show clinical signs of disease at birth (Figure 36). However, the majority of infants severely affected at birth die. Infected babies who do not have clinical signs of disease excrete the virus in the urine for several years and serve as a source of infection. This has special relevance for the pregnant woman who works in a nursery and comes into contact with babies and toddlers. Neurological features which may be present at birth or subsequently develop include microcephaly, cerebral calcifications and choroidoretinitis. Mental and motor retardation is very common in infants who had signs of neurological involvement in the neonatal period.

Rubella Virus

Approximately 0.1 to 2.5 per cent of women acquire primary rubella infection during pregnancy. The incidence of congenital infection in liveborn babies is about 0.07 to 0.7 per cent, increasing to almost 3.0 per cent during epidemics. Spontaneous abortion may result from rubella infection, although the incidence is unknown. Stillbirth and premature delivery are uncommon. Unlike other fetal infections it is certain that an embryopathy occurs, and the risk is related to the age of the fetus when infected. The incidence of embryopathy recognisable at or after birth is 30 to 40 per cent in first trimester infections. When rubella occurs in the first four weeks of pregnancy defects are frequently multiple and the incidence is 50 to 60 per cent. There is probably some risk of fetal damage up to 24 weeks gestation. The results may not be apparent until several years after birth when subtle defects, principally of hearing, become apparent (Hardy *et al.* 1969).

There is a high mortality in those babies who have signs of acute disease, particularly thrombocytopenia, at birth. Neurological abnormalities, including microcephaly or hydrocephaly and convulsions, may be present at birth or subsequently develop. One interesting feature of intra-uterine rubella infection which has immunological implications is that babies may develop 'late onset disease' from three months to one year. The clinical features include skin lesions and a generalised pulmonary disease. The continuum of damage which may result from intrauterine rubella infection makes assessment of the long-term prognosis difficult. Normal educational development is very unlikely when deafness and bilateral cataracts are present.

Toxoplasma gondii

This small protozoan has a worldwide distribution. The parasite is thought to be transmitted to humans from animal reservoirs, particularly dog faeces, but in many parts of the world the eating of uncooked meat is probably an important route of transmission. Desmonts and Couvreur (1968) in a prospective Parisian study showed that congenital toxoplasmosis occurred in 36 per cent of the offspring of mothers who acquired the infection in pregnancy, but the proportion of infected babies who were clinically abnormal at birth was small. One recent survey of pregnant women in London suggested that the infection rate in mothers was 0.2 per cent (Bourne and Rouss 1974).

There is little comprehensive information available concerning the incidence of congenital toxoplasmosis in the UK and USA although it is probably less than that of congenital cytomegalovirus or rubella disease but greater than the incidence of congenital syphilis. Clinical features in the newborn period include jaundice, anaemia, thrombocytopenic purpura, hepatosplenomegaly, choroidoretinitis, microcephaly, hydrocephaly and cerebral calcifications. The precise role of fetal infection in the later development of neurological abnormalities such as convulsions, mental subnormality and motor impairment is unknown.

Bacterial Infections

Virtually any bacterial organism may infect the fetus. Transplacental passage is responsible for fetal infection with *Treponema pallidum* and *Mycobacterium tuberculosis*. Congenital syphilis is uncommon in the UK (less than 30 cases per annum) and USA and congenital tuberculosis is very rare. In the presence of maternal septicaemia, transplacental spread of bacteria to the fetus may occur. Ascending spread from the birth canal probably occurs more frequently than transplacental passage in the case of bacterial infections. Although the incidence of placental inflammation caused by ascending infection may be as high as 50 per cent when the membranes have been ruptured for longer than 24 hours, it should be remembered that ascending bacterial infection can occur through intact membranes. Placental infection is invariably associated with the presence of organisms in the amniotic fluid and there is a positive correlation between fetal bacteraemia and placental infection. However, only a minority of newborn babies with a positive blood culture based on umbilical venous blood samples develop clinical evidence of infection. The bacteria responsible for ascending infection include those which are resident in the mother's bowel and contaminate the vagina and perineum (Table 14). The effects of intrauterine bacterial infections are summarised in Table 15. *Listeria monocytogenes* and *Vibrio fetus* infections have been implicated as a cause of spontaneous abortion. It is not surprising that neonatal pneumonia is the most common acute clinical manifestation of intrauterine bacterial infection when one considers the anatomical continuity between the fetal lung and amniotic cavity. Group B streptococcal infection is a prominent cause.

Infection Acquired During Passage through the Birth Canal

The dividing line between infection acquired as a result of ascending spread and that acquired during passage through the birth canal is blurred. Similar organisms often use both routes of infection (Table 14). The most common manifestation of *Candida albicans* infection is oral thrush. Once the fungus is present in the alimentary tract secondary invasion of all types of napkin area eruptions may occur. *Neisseria gonorrhoeae*, *Mycoplasma pneumoniae* and the TRIC agent may each cause purulent conjunctivitis. Maternal herpetic vulvovaginitis exposes the fetus to herpes simplex during delivery. The effect on the baby may be inapparent or he may develop a mild infection with a few vesicular skin lesions. Spontaneous recovery usually occurs but in some cases a severe, usually fatal disease develops which involves the central nervous system.

The special implications of infection acquired before or during birth may not always be appreciated by the medical attendant because of the diverse nature of signs and symptoms which may be present at birth. Some clues to the presence of infection acquired before or during birth are shown in Table 16.

Postnatal Infection

The skin of the newborn baby becomes colonised at de-

Table 15. The effects of fetal bacterial infection.

Abortion
Stillbirth
Premature delivery

Signs of infection manifesting at birth or within three days:

   Pneumonia
   Septicaemia
   Meningitis
   Pyelonephritis
   Gastroenteritis
   Osteitis, septic arthritis
   Otitis media
   Conjunctivitis
   Omphalitis
   Skin infection

Table 16. Clues to the diagnosis of intrauterine infection.

Unexplained maternal illness during pregnancy, particularly the presence of fever or rash.

Membrane rupture/delivery interval of more than 24 hours.

Maternal fever immediately before, during or after labour.

Abnormal maternal vaginal discharge immediately before, during or after labour.

Signs and symptoms of infection in baby that are present at birth or within three days.

Small for dates baby.

Congenital malformation.

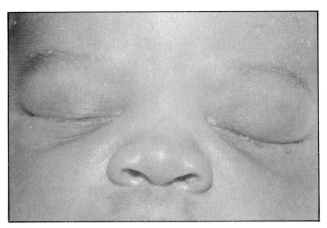

Figure 37. *Severe purulent conjunctivitis. The full extent of the infection may not be appreciated if the eyelids are closed. Note the swelling and erythema of the left eyelid.*

livery with organisms from the maternal vagina. The nose, throat, umbilicus and rectum become colonised during the first few days of life. The principal organisms responsible for disease in the newborn are *Staphylococcus aureus* and Gram-negative bacilli, and any organ-system of the body may be involved. A superficial infection may rapidly spread to deeper tissues and once septicaemia has occurred multiple sites of infection are to be expected. The rapidity of spread in untreated cases underlines the importance of the early recognition of sepsis in the neonate.

Recognition of Sepsis

Even superficial infection may be overlooked on casual examination. For example, the full extent of purulent conjunctivitis is often not appreciated when the baby's eyelids are closed (Figure 37) and paronychia can also be easily overlooked if the baby is examined without removing his mittens and socks.

Staphylococcal skin sepsis may be associated with widely differing skin lesions (Figure 38). Umbilical sepsis has special relevance because the umbilical cord stump is an excellent culture medium and gives organisms an easy mode of entry to the bloodstream. A moist stump is not necessarily infected, and of greater importance is the presence of periumbilical erythema and a foul smell.

The diagnosis of infection in deep tissues requires a high index of suspicion on the part of medical and nursing personnel. The important infections are septicaemia, meningitis, pneumonia, gastroenteritis, pyelonephritis, osteitis, arthritis and otitis media. The neonate usually presents with nonspecific signs and symptoms rather than features which point to involvement of a particular organ-system (Table 17). The nurse or mother who is in frequent contact with the baby is usually the first to notice a subtle change in the baby's pattern of behaviour. Such warnings must not go unheeded merely because the baby's body temperature is normal. The neonate with severe sepsis may have a sub-normal, normal, or raised body temperature. *Meningitis* does not present with neck stiffness and

convulsions, which are very late signs of the disease in the neonatal period. A normal anterior fontanelle is the usual finding early in the course of the disease. *Pneumonia* may occur with minimal or absent respiratory signs. *Gastro-enteritis* may present with abdominal distension and vomiting without the frequent passage of loose stools. Severe fluid and electrolyte loss commonly occurs into the lumen of the bowel and in the absence of diarrhoea the full extent of the losses may not be appreciated.

Pyelonephritis is equally common in males and females in the neonatal period, and may be associated with struc-

Figure 38. *Staphylococcal skin sepsis presenting as a) an exfoliative lesion, and b) vesicular lesion.*

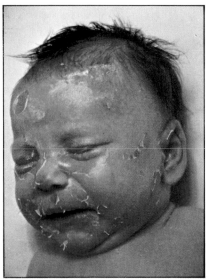

a

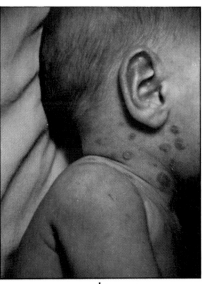

b

Table 17. Nonspecific signs and symptoms of neonatal infection.

Symptoms	Signs
'Not doing well'	Jaundice
Reluctance to feed	Abdominal distension
Lethargy	Unstable body temperature
Vomiting	Mild splenomegaly
Diarrhoea	Bilateral renal enlargement
Irritability	Purpuric skin rash
Cyanotic or apnoeic attacks	
Hypoglycaemia	

Table 18. Aids in the diagnosis of congenital or acquired infection.

Placenta	—histology and culture
Amniotic fluid	—microscopy and culture
Maternal vaginal swab	—microscopy and culture
Cord blood	—IgM and serology as indicated
Baby's blood	Serial IgM estimations and serology as indicated / Bacterial or viral culture / White cell count and differential / Examination of blood film
urine / CSF	microscopy and culture
stools / throat swab / nose swab / umbilical swab / Chest X-ray	culture

Note. Any baby with nonspecific signs of infection must have blood, urine, CSF and stool cultures in addition to superficial swab cultures.

tural malformation of the urinary tract. The abdomen should be carefully examined for signs of kidney or bladder enlargement. The urinary stream should be observed particularly in male babies who are prone to urinary obstruction from posterior urethral valves. A normal urinary stream does not exclude the presence of urethral valves but a dribbling stream in a male baby with a urinary tract infection strongly supports the diagnosis. *Osteitis* and *septic arthritis,* like other deep infections, may present with lethargy and failure to feed. However, excessive crying may occur when the baby is handled because of a painful limb and diminished spontaneous movement of the limb is an important sign. A baby with 'cellulitis' who also has nonspecific signs and symptoms of infection is probably suffering from osteitis or septic arthritis. In *septicaemia,* jaundice, splenomegaly and slight bilateral renal enlargement occur. *Otitis media* certainly does occur in the neonatal period (McLellan *et al.* 1962) and auroscopic examination should be made in all neonates with nonspecific signs or symptoms of sepsis.

Investigation of Infection

Aids in the diagnosis of infection are summarised in Table 18. When it is suspected at birth that infection was acquired *in utero,* the placenta should be saved for histological examination and culture, a specimen of cord blood taken for serological study and a vaginal swab taken from the mother for culture. A cord blood IgM concentration greater then 20 mg per cent supports the diagnosis of intrauterine infection. When a congenital non-bacterial infection is suspected the laboratory should be informed at once because the studies made are determined by the local facilities. In the presence of serious bacterial infection, unduly heavy colonisation of the throat, nose and umbilicus is common. Any ill baby with nonspecific signs of infection should have specimens of peripheral venous blood, cerebrospinal fluid, urine and faeces cultured without delay. A total neutrophil count above 6,900 per mm³ or below 1,400 per mm³ after 72 hours of age supports the diagnosis of bacterial infection as does a metamyelocyte count greater than 500 per mm³ (Xanthou 1970).

Treatment

A detailed review of the management of infection in the neonate is beyond the scope of this chapter, but certain principles deserve special mention. There is little to be gained from the prophylactic use of antibiotics in the neonatal period. However, antibiotics should be readily administered at the slightest suspicion that bacterial sepsis is present. Treatment should be started immediately after the relevant specimens have been taken for culture. The antibiotic used may have to be modified in the light of the subsequent bacteriological report. The initial choice of antibiotic depends on many factors, including knowledge of the bacterial flora to which the baby has been exposed prior to the development of symptoms. A combination of antibiotics which provide a wide spectrum of antibacterial action is preferable (for example, penicillin and gentamicin). The intramuscular rather than the oral route should be used during the first two weeks of life because of uncertain absorption from the gastrointestinal tract. The suggested dosage of certain antibiotics is shown in Table 20. The duration of treatment for proven bloodstream infection should be at least 10 days. Neonates with meningitis require treatment for at least three weeks and those with osteitis, septic arthritis or pyelonephritis require treatment for six weeks.

Purulent conjunctivitis must be treated energetically with antibacterial eye drops every 15 minutes or so for the first hour, gradually reducing the frequency as the discharge clears. When gonococcal infection is suspected penicillin drops (2,500 units per ml) should be used together with systemic benzylpenicillin. Sulphacetamide eye drops (10 per cent) may be used for non-gonococcal eye infections pending the results of the eye swab culture.

Table 19. Suggested dosages of antibacterial drugs.

Drug	Single intramuscular dose[3]	Oral dose/24 hours
Cephaloridine[1] (Ceporin)	15 mg/kg	
Colistin (Colomycin)	25,000 u/kg (not exceeding 75,000 u/kg/day)	125,000 u/kg
Erythromycin (Erythrocin, Erythromid, Erythroped)	5 mg/kg	25 mg/kg
Gentamicin[1] (Cidomycin, Genticin)	3 mg/kg initial dose 2 mg/kg subsequent doses	
Kanamycin[2] (Kannasyn, Kantrex)	5–7 mg/kg	
Neomycin (Neomin, Nivemycin)	2.5 mg/kg	50 mg/kg
Benzylpenicillin (Crystapen, Eskacillin 100, Falapen, Solupen)	15,000 u/kg	40,000 u/kg
Ampicillin (Penbritin)	25 mg/kg	60 mg/kg
Carbenicillin (Pyopen)	100 mg/kg	
Cloxacillin (Orbenin)	12.5 mg/kg	30 mg/kg
Methicillin (Celbenin)	20 mg/kg	
Polymyxin methane sulphonate	20,000 u/kg (not exceeding 40,000 u/kg/day)	
Streptomycin[2] (Orastrep)	7–10 mg/kg	20 mg/kg
Sulphadimidine (Sulphamethazine)	7.5 mg/kg	50 mg/kg

Modified from Davies *et al.* (1972), except for gentamicin dose (Milner *et al.* 1972).
[1]Need not be given more than 8-hourly IM.
[2]Need not be given more than 12-hourly IM.
[3]Intramuscular dose: for term infants the above doses should be given 8-hourly for the first two weeks and 6-hourly thereafter unless otherwise shown. For premature infants give 12-hourly in the first week of life, 8-hourly between one and four weeks and 6-hourly if over four weeks unless otherwise shown.

Table 20. Measures to reduce the incidence of infection in the neonatal nursery.

The policy of feeding babies with fresh human milk which has many antibacterial properties.

Scrupulous hand washing before and after handling each baby.

The use of aseptic techniques for procedures such as umbilical vessel catheterisation, intubation, etc.

Sterilisation and careful supervision of equipment such as incubators and mechanical ventilators, etc.

Supervision of well-recognised 'germ traps', for example washbasins and sinks.

Treatment of the skin and umbilicus of the newborn with an appropriate antibacterial preparation, so reducing the spread of staphylococcal organisms.

Early diagnosis and treatment of neonatal infection, so reducing the opportunity for serious cross infection.

Prevention of Infection

Examples of specific prophylactic measures to reduce the incidence of congenital infection are poliovirus and rubella virus immunisation, which reduce the number of pregnant women exposed to primary infection. A major change in policy with respect to the prevention of cross infection in newborn nurseries has occurred in the past 10 to 15 years. Allowing visitors to the nursery is not associated with an increased incidence of neonatal infection, and the wearing of gowns and masks does not significantly contribute to the safety of neonates. The single most important measure in the prevention of infection in the newborn nursery is scrupulous hand washing. A summary of important measures to reduce the incidence of neonatal infection is shown in Table 20.

References

Bourne, G. L. and Rouss, C. F., cited by Fleck, D. G. in *Intra-Uterine Infections,* p. 46, Associated Scientific Publishers, Amsterdam, 1974.

Davies, P. A., Robinson, R. J., Scopes, J. W., Tizard, J. P. M. and Wigglesworth, J. S., *Medical Care of Newborn Babies*, p. 170, Spastics International Medical Publications, William Heinemann Ltd., London, 1972.

Desmonts, G. and Couvreur, J., cited by Remington, J. S. in *Prenatal Infections*, p. 9, Georg Thieme, Stuttgart, 1968.

Hardy, J. B., McCracken, G. H., Gilkeston, M. R. and Sever, J. L., *JAMA*, 1969, **207**, 2414.

McLellan, M. S., Strong, J. P., Johnson, O. R. and Dent, J. H., *J. Pediat.* 1962, **61**, 53.

Milner, R. D. G., Ross, J., Froud, D. J. R. and Davis, J. A., *Arch. Dis. Childh.*, 1972, **47**, 927.

Xanthou, M., *Arch. Dis. Childh.*, 1970, **45**, 242.

Further Reading

Alford, C. A. Jr., *Pediat. Clin. N. Amer*, 1971, **18**, 99.

Ledger, W. J. (Ed.), Infectious diseases in perinatology. In : *Seminars in Perinatology*, 1977, **1**, 1–101, Grune and Stratton, New York.

7. Jaundice

ABOUT 85 per cent of the circulating unconjugated bilirubin pool is formed from the breakdown of haemoglobin, and the remainder from the catabolism of other haem-containing pigments.

One gram of haemoglobin yields 35 mg of unconjugated bilirubin which circulates bound to albumin. In fetal life unconjugated bilirubin is cleared into the maternal circulation by the placenta. After birth, unconjugated bilirubin is transported to the liver, and within the hepatocyte the enzyme glucuronyl transferase conjugates bilirubin with glucuronic acid. Conjugated bilirubin is excreted into the biliary tree and thence into the gut lumen, where the enzyme β-glucuronidase hydrolyses a proportion of the bilirubin to the unconjugated type, which is reabsorbed into the circulation bound to albumin and undergoes hepatic clearance once again (the enterohepatic circulation) (Figure 39). The remaining conjugated bilirubin in the gut lumen is excreted in the stools as stercobilinogen, or absorbed by the circulation and excreted in the urine as urobilinogen.

Neonatal jaundice is usually associated with a raised blood level of unconjugated bilirubin which produces the characteristic golden-yellow discoloration of the baby's skin. Rarely, a significant proportion of the circulating bilirubin is of the conjugated type giving a green-yellow tinge to the skin. The implications of neonatal jaundice are: first, it may indicate the presence of an underlying disease requiring specific treatment; second, unconjugated bilirubin that is 'free' or unbound to albumin is lipid-soluble and toxic to the CNS.

Physiological Jaundice

The concept of physiological jaundice is a useful one because it describes a type of jaundice which is very common, apparently harmless and does not require laboratory investigation. It is characterised by its appearance in a well baby after the first 48 hours of life, reaching a peak by about the fourth day and disappearing within seven to ten days. The peak blood level of bilirubin, which is unconjugated, is below 10 to 12 mg per cent[1]. The cause of the jaundice is not entirely understood. Multiple factors undoubtedly contribute to the aetiology (Table 21). In the following circumstances jaundice should never be accepted as physiological, and a search for the cause must be made:

Table 21. Factors which contribute to physiological jaundice in the newborn.

Shortened red blood cell lifespan (90 days).
Catabolism of non-haem pigment is substantial, contributing to 15 to 20 per cent of the unconjugated bilirubin pool.
Reduced liver perfusion (patency of ductus venosus).
Impaired uptake of bilirubin by hepatocyte.
Transient deficiency of enzymes involved in bilirubin conjugation.
Enterohepatic circulation of bilirubin.

1. An unwell baby.

2. Visible jaundice present in the first 24 hours of life.

3. Persistent jaundice beyond the tenth day of life.

4. Recurrence of jaundice after an initial improvement.

5. Total bilirubin level > 12 mg per cent or conjugated fraction > 2.0 mg per cent.

Pathological Jaundice

To appreciate the various aetiologies of pathological jaundice (see Table 22) it is necessary to consider the three mechanisms by which jaundice is produced:

1. Overproduction of bilirubin.

2. Impaired hepatic clearance of bilirubin.

3. Both overproduction and impaired hepatic clearance.

The plasma bilirubin concentration depends on a balance between bilirubin formation and hepatic clearance. In the face of impaired hepatic clearance unconjugated bilirubin accumulates in the plasma, if the hepatic defect is proximal to the point at which bilirubin conjugation occurs. If impaired hepatic clearance occurs beyond the stage at which bilirubin conjugation occurs, then the conjugated pigment accumulates in the plasma.

Overproduction of Bilirubin

Haemolytic Disease

Jaundice occurring within the first 24 hours of life is usually caused by haemolytic disease. Maternal–fetal

---

[1]To convert SI units, see footnote on page 26.

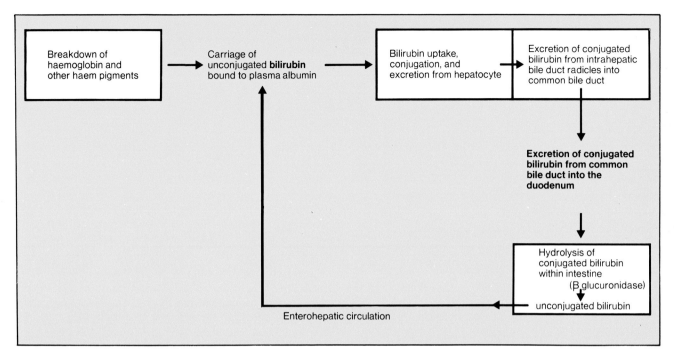

Figure 39. *The formation and hepatic clearance of bilirubin. The enterohepatic circulation.*

blood group incompatibility accounts for most cases of haemolytic disease. ABO incompatibility is the most common cause, but in terms of severity, Rh incompatibility is the most important. Hereditary spherocytosis is not rare and, although inherited as an autosomal dominant, the disease may not be demonstrable in either parent in 10 to 25 per cent of cases (Young 1955).

Jaundice of early onset in babies of people of Mediterranean or African origin may be associated with haemolytic disorders involving red-cell enzyme defects or haemoglobinopathies. Any of the haemolytic disorders in the neonatal period may cause severe jaundice and a risk of kernicterus, but a uniform clinical picture is not to be expected. Pallor and hepatosplenomegaly are usually present in severe Rh haemolytic disease but are inconstant findings in ABO incompatibility and hereditary spherocytosis.

The laboratory investigations which are helpful in the diagnosis of haemolytic jaundice are shown in Table 23. In ABO incompatibility and hereditary spherocytosis the haemoglobin level may be normal or only slightly reduced in spite of marked jaundice. The direct Coombs' test is positive in Rh disease, but usually negative in ABO incompatibility. In the latter disease the mother is blood group O and the baby A or B, and the presence of high titres of anti-A or anti-B haemolysins in maternal or baby blood suggests the diagnosis. After the third day of life a reticulocyte count of more than six per cent suggests the presence of a haemolytic process. A blood smear should be examined by a haematologist who has experience in interpreting blood films of newborn babies. The presence of microspherocytes, polychromasia and anisocytosis are all suggestive of a haemolytic process.

Heinz bodies and bizarre-shaped red cells may be a clue to the presence of one of the rarer red cell abnormalities as a cause of haemolytic disease.

Extravasation of Blood

Dangerously high levels of circulating bilirubin requiring multiple exchange transfusions may occur as a result of the breakdown of blood which has become extravasated into various sites, for instance intracranial haemorrhage, bruising, cephalhaematoma. Bruising is a common cause of jaundice, particularly in premature babies and those born by the breech. Even in the absence of external bruising, significant quantities of blood may become extravasated between the layers of the gluteal muscles in breech deliveries (Ralis 1975). The onset of jaundice is usually after 48 hours.

Polycythaemia

Jaundice resulting from polycythaemia usually occurs after the first 48 hours of life. The venous packed-cell volume is greater than 70 per cent. The full extent of the jaundice may not be initially appreciated because of the baby's plethoric appearance. When clinically assessing the degree of jaundice the skin should be blanched by finger compression and the colour observed immediately after releasing the finger. Some conditions associated with neonatal polycythaemia are shown in Table 22.

Increased Enterohepatic Circulation

Any condition associated with intestinal stasis, including congenital obstruction, may lead to an increased enterohepatic circulation. Presumably under these circumstances conjugated bilirubin within the bowel lumen has a greater opportunity to be hydrolysed by β-glucuronidase, yielding unconjugated bilirubin. An additional factor in the mechanism of the jaundice concerns the role played by the bacterial flora of the bowel. Beyond the immediate newborn period, when the bowel flora is established, conjugated bilirubin in the bowel is broken down to stercobilinogen. The presence of a high congenital gut obstruction delays bacterial colonisation of the bowel and thereby allows the continued hydrolysis of conjugated bilirubin to the unconjugated form. An increased entero-hepatic circulation alone does not give rise to severe jaundice but may well aggravate jaundice resulting from some other cause.

Impaired Hepatic Clearance of Bilirubin

A high index of suspicion is required for the diagnosis of jaundice associated with impaired hepatic clearance of bilirubin. It should be suspected in the absence of a haemolytic process, extravasation of blood, or polycy-thaemia when the jaundice is beyond 'physiological' limits (plasma bilirubin >10 to 12 mg per cent), persists for longer than ten days or is associated with the presence of significant amounts of conjugated bilirubin in the plasma (>2 mg per cent).

Hypothyroidism

Jaundice associated with raised levels of unconjugated bilirubin which persist after ten days is a feature of many babies with congenital hypothyroidism. It is not clear whether the primary defect is that of bilirubin uptake by the hepatocyte, or conjugation. The jaundice is not usually of such severity as to require exchange transfu-sion. Associated clinical features of hypothyroidism may coexist, including the characteristic facial appearance, lethargy and constipation. However, prolonged jaundice is often the only clinical clue to the diagnosis of hypo-thyroidism. All babies with prolonged and persistent jaundice should have the appropriate laboratory tests of thyroid function (blood TSH, T_4, T_3, and cholesterol).

Inborn Errors of Metabolism

Galactosaemia and certain inborn errors of amino-acid metabolism (tyrosinosis, hypermethioninaemia) are as-sociated with raised levels of unconjugated bilirubin in the blood during the first week of life, caused either by impaired uptake of bilirubin by the hepatocyte, defective conjugation, or both. Subsequently, hepatic damage occurs and impaired transport of conjugated bilirubin from the liver leads to the accumulation of significant amounts of conjugated bilirubin in the bloodstream. In galactosaemia, additional clinical features that may be present include vomiting, failure to thrive, hepatomegaly, haemorrhagic manifestations and the development of cataracts.

Babies who are jaundiced in association with distur-bances of amino-acid metabolism are usually very ill. Vomiting, dehydration, acidosis and hypoglycaemia may be prominent features. A definitive diagnosis in jaundice associated with inborn errors of metabolism is more likely to be achieved by liaison with a suitably equipped metabolic laboratory. However, an important clue to the diagnosis of galactosaemia may be obtained by ward

Table 22. Causes of pathological jaundice.

Overproduction of bilirubin	Impaired hepatic clearance of bilirubin	Mixed

1. Haemolytic disease
  a) Fetomaternal blood group incompatibility (ABO, rhesus, etc.)
  b) Hereditary spherocytosis
  c) Red cell enzyme defects (G6PD, pyruvate kinase, etc.)
  d) Haemoglobinopathies
	1. Congenital hypothyroidism
	
	2. Inborn errors of metabolism
	  a) Galactosaemia
	  b) Tyrosinosis, hypermethioninaemia
		1. Prematurity
		
		2. Postnatal sepsis
		
		3. Neonatal hepatitis
		  a) Rubella virus
		  b) Cytomegalovirus
		  c) *Toxoplasma gondii*
		  d) Herpes simplex
		  e) *Treponema pallidum*

2. Extravasation of blood
  a) External bruising, haematomata, etc.
  b) Internal haemorrhage
	3. Breast milk jaundice
	
	4. Crigler–Najjar syndrome	

3. Polycythaemia
  a) Maternofetal, twin-twin transfusion
  b) Delayed clamping of cord
  c) Small-for-dates babies
  d) Infants of diabetic mothers
  e) Neonatal thyrotoxicosis
  f) Congenital adrenal hyperplasia
  g) Down's syndrome
	5. Obstructive jaundice
	  a) Congenital biliary atresia
	  b) Choledochal cyst
	  c) Cystic fibrosis
	  d) α_1 antitrypsin deficiency	

4. Increased enterohepatic circulation
  a) Paralytic ileus
  b) Poor fluid intake
  c) Congenital gut obstruction		

testing of the patient's urine. A significant amount of galactose in the urine is associated with a positive 'Clinitest' confirming the presence of reducing substances, and a negative 'Clinistix', indicating that the offending reducing substance is not glucose.

Breast Milk Jaundice

The milk of certain mothers contains a progesterone derivative which inhibits the conjugation of bilirubin. The resulting jaundice develops on about the third day and usually persists for several weeks. Bilirubin levels above 12 mg per cent are quite common. The diagnosis may be confirmed by observing the effect of the mother's milk on bilirubin conjugation in an *in vitro* system (e.g. rat liver slices). There are very few centres that undertake such measurements. It may be argued that knowing whether or not there is an 'inhibitor' in the mother's milk rarely influences clinical practice.

In most cases a gradual reduction in the level of serum bilirubin occurs in spite of the continuation of breast feeding. Provided the levels of bilirubin are carefully monitored, the advantages of breast feeding usually outweigh the hazards of hyperbilirubinaemia. If the serum bilirubin approaches 'toxic' levels (say > 20 mg per cent in an otherwise well term baby), breast feeding should be temporarily discontinued and appropriate measures taken to reduce the bilirubin level (see below). It is likely that in many cases so-called breast-milk jaundice is associated with a poor fluid intake and hypoperistalsis leading to an increased enterohepatic circulation.

Crigler–Najjar Syndrome

The Crigler–Najjar syndrome is a rare familial condition inherited as an autosomal recessive and associated with a deficiency of glucuronyl transferase in the hepatocyte. In severe forms dangerous high levels of unconjugated bilirubin accumulate in the blood and there is a very real risk of kernicterus. Although the jaundice is persistent, it is interesting that the serum bilirubin level tends to become stabilised after the newborn period.

Obstructive Jaundice

Impaired transport of bilirubin beyond the stage at which conjugation occurs is associated with the accumulation of conjugated bilirubin in the blood (> 2 mg per cent). The conditions associated with obstructive jaundice (Table 22) usually present with jaundice just beyond the neonatal period but occasionally jaundice is present as early as the third week (Figure 40). It is usually very difficult to distinguish one type of obstructive jaundice from another clinically. Furthermore, there is usually an associated rise of unconjugated bilirubin in the blood because of defective hepatic transport before the stage of conjugation. These types of jaundice are liable to be confused with the jaundice of certain intrauterine infections which cause hepatitis. Indeed it is possible that certain types of intrahepatic biliary atresia represent the end result of intrauterine hepatitis of infective origin. A mass in the right upper zone of the abdomen can sometimes be

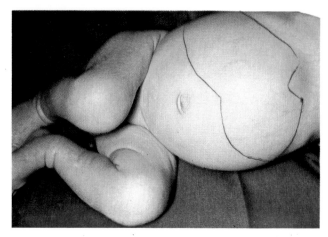

Figure 40. *A three-week-old baby with hepatomegaly and jaundice associated with a high level of serum conjugated bilirubin. Subsequent laparotomy revealed atresia of the extrahepatic bile ducts.*

Figure 41. *An ill neonate with* E. coli *septicaemia. The presenting signs 24 hours previously were jaundice, lethargy and reluctance to feed.*

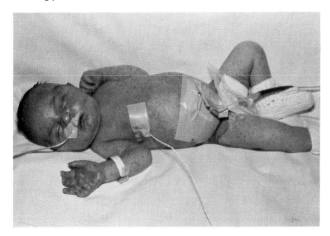

felt in babies who have a choledochal cyst.

Babies with cystic fibrosis may have a history of intestinal obstruction associated with meconium ileus, and a raised sweat sodium concentration confirms the diagnosis. Deficiency of α_1 antitrypsin activity in the serum is associated with chronic pulmonary disease in adolescence and adulthood. Neonates have been described with the enzyme deficiency in association with an obstructive jaundice caused by hepatitis. The precise relationship of α_1 antitrypsin deficiency to neonatal liver disease, ongoing liver disease (chronic hepatitis, cirrhosis) and the pulmonary lesion is not known.

Combined Overproduction and Impaired Hepatic Clearance of Bilirubin

Prematurity

Jaundice of prematurity is usually attributed to factors associated with 'physiological jaundice', particularly a deficiency of glucuronyl transferase, being exaggerated in the premature baby. This is a dangerous assumption because prematurity itself is a pathological state, and what is physiological for the mature neonate outside the womb may be pathological for the baby whose rightful place is inside the womb. Multiple factors contribute to the aetiology of jaundice of prematurity. Although hepatic clearance of unconjugated bilirubin is impaired, contributory factors include:

1. Persistent patency of ductus venosus, diverting blood away from the liver.

2. Bruising.

3. Hypoperistalsis and an increased enterohepatic circulation.

Postnatal Sepsis

The prudent neonatologist does not believe that mild or moderate jaundice *per se* causes lethargy and reluctance to feed. Sepsis (Figure 41) causes lethargy, reluctance to feed and jaundice! Certain bacteria produce haemolysins which reduce red-cell survival. An ill baby with sepsis may have a poor fluid intake, hypoperistalsis and an increased enterohepatic circulation. Liver uptake and conjugation of the excess load of bilirubin is probably impaired in ill babies. Finally, impaired hepatic clearance of conjugated bilirubin may lead to a slight rise of serum conjugated bilirubin.

Neonatal Hepatitis

Neonatal hepatitis may present with hepatosplenomegaly, anaemia and purpura in addition to jaundice. The inflammatory lesion of the liver impairs the clearance of conjugated bilirubin and up to 50 per cent of the total serum bilirubin may be the conjugated type. Associated haemolysis and haemorrhage lead to an overproduction of unconjugated bilirubin.

A summary of the investigations that are helpful in the diagnosis of pathological jaundice is shown in Table 23.

Bilirubin Toxicity

Kernicterus is the immediate clinical manifestation of bilirubin toxicity. The initial signs are those of CNS depression with hypotonia, diminished or incomplete Moro reflex, difficulty in feeding and vomiting. Subsequently the baby becomes irritable with a shrill cry, hypertonia, opisthotonic posturing, downward deviation of the eyes and convulsions. Later clinical manifestations in surviving infants include cerebral palsy of the athetoid type, sensorineural deafness and mental retardation. Hyperbilirubinaemia in the newborn period, not resulting in overt kernicterus, may be associated with signs of 'minimal brain damage' in later childhood. Once signs of bilirubin toxicity are manifest the situation is irreversible. The problem is the recognition of the neonate who has hyperbilirubinaemia of such a degree that there is a high risk of CNS damage.

Albumin-bound unconjugated bilirubin is harmless, but

Table 23. Some laboratory investigations helpful in establishing the aetiology of pathological jaundice.

1. Suspected haemolytic jaundice
    a) Haemoglobin, haematocrit
    b) Blood group of mother and baby
    c) Direct Coombs' test
    d) Reticulocyte count
    e) Blood film
    f) If indicated: red blood cell enzyme studies
                    haemoglobin electrophoresis
                    osmotic fragility of red blood cells
                    titre of anti-A or anti-B haemolysins
                      in maternal or baby blood
2. Non-haemolytic jaundice
    a) Total white cell count and differential
    b) Serum IgM
    c) Bacterial cultures (superficial, blood, urine, CSF)
    d) 'Clinitest' and 'Clinistix'
    e) If indicated: viral culture (throat swab, urine,
                      blood)
                    serum transaminases and alkaline
                      phosphatase
                    thyroid function tests
                    plasma and urinary amino acids
                    serum α_1 antitrypsin
                    sweat sodium concentration

free unconjugated bilirubin, which is lipid-soluble and readily diffuses into brain-cell membranes, is toxic. Kernicterus is associated with yellow staining of the basal ganglia and hippocampus on post-mortem examination of the brain. Measurements of serum bilirubin in common use do not distinguish between the free and bound fraction. In the presence of low serum albumin levels, which may occur in premature babies, there are fewer binding sites available for bilirubin. It may, therefore, appear in the plasma in the free form in the face of total serum bilirubin concentrations which are only moderately raised. Certain drugs and chemicals displace bilirubin from albumin-binding sites, e.g. salicylates, sulphonamides, benzoates and free fatty acids. Acidaemia reduces the affinity of bilirubin for albumin.

A future development will be the widespread use of methods for assessing the reserve binding power of albumin for bilirubin, which will enable more accurate prediction of impending bilirubin toxicity. For the present it is reasonable to assume that in an otherwise well term baby a concentration of unconjugated bilirubin > 20 mg per cent is potentially toxic and warrants treatment. In an otherwise well premature baby concentrations > 15 mg per cent may be toxic. Regardless of maturity the occurrence of asphyxia, cerebral trauma, hypoxia, acidosis and sepsis significantly increases the risk of bilirubin encephalopathy at a given serum bilirubin concentration.

Treatment of Hyperbilirubinaemia

Exchange Transfusion

Exchange transfusion is performed when the serum bilirubin approaches toxic levels. The mortality from the

Table 24. Complications associated with exchange transfusion.

Bacteraemia, viraemia
Cardiac failure or sudden cardiac arrest
a) Volume overload
b) Arrhythmias
c) Uncertain aetiology
Electrolyte disturbances
a) Hyperkalaemia
b) Hypocalcaemia
c) Acidosis
Embolic phenomena
a) Air
b) Thrombus
Hypothermia
Hypoglycaemia
Necrotising enterocolitis

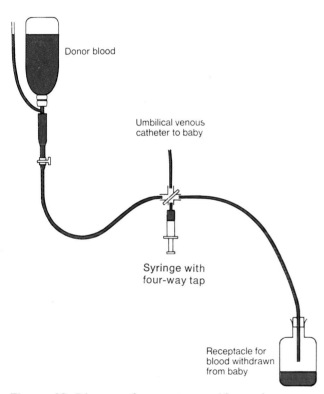

Figure 42. *Diagram of apparatus used for exchange transfusion.*

procedure in experienced hands is less than one per cent. The complications are shown in Table 24. The implications of the choice of donor blood are outside the scope of this chapter beyond the fact that the blood should be as fresh as possible and certainly not more than four days old.

The exchange is usually performed via an umbilical venous catheter attached to a four-way tap. The limbs of the tap are connected to a 20 ml syringe, the donor blood supply and a receptacle for blood removed from the baby (Figure 42). Ten to 20 ml aliquots of blood are removed from the baby and replaced by donor blood. The total volume of blood exchanged is 180 ml per kg body weight, which is about twice the baby's blood volume. This usually results in a 50 per cent reduction in the serum bilirubin concentration.

Phototherapy

When light of wavelength 400 to 500 nm is shone directly onto the skin of jaundiced babies, the unconjugated bilirubin circulating in the skin capillaries is photo-oxidised to apparently harmless derivatives. This is associated with a reduction in the serum bilirubin concentration and a fading of the jaundice.

Phototherapy units consisting of white or blue lamps are used. The treatment may be used prophylactically to prevent or slow down the rise of serum bilirubin in some types of non-haemolytic jaundice, or as an adjunct to exchange transfusion in haemolytic jaundice. Long-term side-effects attributed to phototherapy have not been reported. Some immediate side-effects are shown in Table 25.

Drugs

Several drugs, including phenobarbitone, stimulate the production of glucuronyl transferase in the liver of the fetus and newborn. Phenobarbitone is sometimes used prophylactically with varying degrees of success in premature babies who have slight or moderate jaundice, or in babies who are badly bruised at birth and who may be expected to develop hyperbilirubinaemia.

Table 25. Some immediate complications of phototherapy.

Retinal damage has been demonstrated in piglets exposed to artificial light in the newborn period. The eyes of the baby should be shielded from the light with a bandage or other eye shield.

The eye bandage may slip over the nostrils causing nasal obstruction.

Conjunctivitis (infective or traumatic) from unsupervised use of eye shields.

Loose stools.

Increased insensible water loss.

Hypothermia (naked baby in cool room) or hyperthermia if there is a high output of radiant heat from phototherapy unit.

Diffuse macular rash.

Bronze discoloration of skin.

Less physical contact between mother and baby particularly when treatment is prolonged.

References

Ralis, Z. A., *Arch. Dis. Child.,* 1975, **50**, 4.
Young, L. E., *Am. J. Med.,* 1955, **18**, 486.

8. Respiratory Problems

RESPIRATORY adaptation to extrauterine life entails more than the establishment of respiration at birth. Ventilation must be such that optimal pulmonary gaseous exchange occurs. There are three common ways in which breathing problems may present:

1. Respiratory distress.
2. Apnoeic attacks.
3. Periodic breathing.

Respiratory Distress

A baby has respiratory distress when two or more of the signs shown in Table 26 are present. In keeping with the neonate's characteristic of responding to diverse diseases with a limited array of physical signs, we are at once handicapped by the fact that signs of respiratory distress may be a reflection of quite different types of pulmonary or even non-pulmonary disease.

Non-Pulmonary Causes of Respiratory Distress

Non-pulmonary causes of respiratory distress are given in Table 27. Acute blood loss and congenital heart disease have been selected for discussion because of the therapeutic importance of making a prompt diagnosis.

Acute Blood Loss

Acute blood loss may present soon after birth, when after a difficult resuscitation the baby remains pale and develops tachycardia, tachypnoea and grunting. The pallor may be attributed to an asphyxial insult and the tachypnoea and grunting may prompt the clinician to focus on the respiratory system. Clues to the correct diagnosis are that the tachypnoea is usually out of proportion to any thoracic-cage retraction, and tachycardia and pallor are prominent features. The peripheral pulses are poor. A metabolic acidosis and low venous haematocrit and haemoglobin level are to be expected. Bleeding from the umbilical cord may be associated with unexpected and unattended home delivery. This should be remembered by the hospital doctor treating a baby who was 'born before arrival' and by the family doctor who may be suddenly called to visit a pale, tachypnoeic and grunting baby.

The restoration of circulating volume is the goal of therapy and the volume expander used (normal saline, plasma, whole blood) depends upon availability. Fresh whole blood is preferable. Circumstances may dictate that uncrossmatched blood from a nearby observer be used. The volume given via the umbilical vein is 20 to 30 ml/kg of the baby's weight and the first 20 to 40 ml is given in about 15 minutes.

Congenital Heart Disease

Certain types of congenital heart disease (CHD) present in the newborn period with signs of respiratory distress of which cyanosis may be a prominent feature (Figure 43). When this occurs a deteriorating course is to be expected. In some lesions, for example transposition of the great vessels, immediate surgical intervention may be lifesaving. Death is inevitable in certain other lesions such as severe hypoplasia of the left ventricle. A high index of suspicion is necessary so that newborn babies suspected of having CHD may be promptly referred to a cardiologist for diagnosis based on the results of cardiac catheterisation.

There is no simple and reliable clinical way of distinguishing respiratory from cardiac causes of respiratory distress in every case. The presence of cyanosis as a

Table 26. Signs of respiratory distress in the newborn.

Tachypnoea (respiratory rate > 60 per min)
Chest-wall retraction on inspiration
Grunting or whining on expiration
Flaring of nostrils
Cyanosis
Use of accessory muscles of respiration

Table 27. Non-pulmonary causes of respiratory distress.

Acute blood loss
Congenital heart disease
Hypothermia
Hyperthermia
Metabolic acidosis
Polycythaemia
Intracranial birth trauma

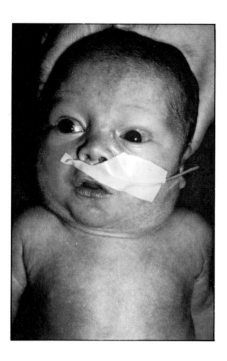

Figure 43. *Marked cyanosis in a newborn baby with congenital heart disease.*

prominent presenting feature, signs of cardiac failure, a heart murmur and clinical or radiological evidence of cardiomegaly all suggest CHD, but there are many diagnostic pitfalls. The following points may be helpful:

1. Consider the possibility of CHD when the clinical history and chest X-ray findings seem out of keeping with a diagnosis of pulmonary disease.

2. Cyanosis in CHD results from a right to left shunt of blood because of an anatomical defect. Cyanosis that disappears when the baby breathes 100 per cent oxygen is not caused by CHD.

3. Do not dismiss the diagnosis of CHD because of the absence of a cardiac murmur or the presence of only a very soft murmur. Severe CHD in the newborn period is more commonly associated with a soft 'insignificant' murmur than a loud one, and often there is no murmur.

4. Life-threatening CHD may not be associated with signs of congestive cardiac failure. However, if heart failure is present, hepatomegaly rather than oedema is a prominent feature. Signs of congestive cardiac failure secondary to a pulmonary disorder are rare in the newborn period.

5. A pale baby with tachycardia, tachypnoea and weak peripheral pulses may have serious CHD (or acute blood loss!).

6. A normal size heart on chest X-ray is often seen in CHD. Particular attention should be paid to the lung fields. Oligaemic or plethoric pulmonary vasculature suggests CHD.

7. The significance of ECG findings of right ventricular hypertrophy is usually difficult to assess in the immediate newborn period. In contrast, left ventricular hypertrophy is always abnormal.

Pulmonary Causes of Respiratory Distress

Aetiological factors in the common respiratory disorders usually operate before or during birth and only occasionally does respiratory disease arise *de novo* solely from a postnatal influence. This concept forms the basis for the diagnosis of many of the common causes of respiratory distress. A careful review of antecedent events, together with a chest X-ray, will in most cases be more helpful than the use of a stethoscope in suggesting the correct diagnosis. Although auscultation of the chest should not be omitted, its role is probably limited to establishing the presence of asymmetrical breath sounds and displacement of the apex beat.

Pulmonary causes of respiratory distress are shown in Table 28. In some disorders (for example, diaphragmatic hernia, tension pneumothorax) the baby's survival is greatly dependent on the promptness of diagnosis. In other circumstances one might initially and safely settle for an undetermined cause, while providing the baby with supportive care of which the most important aspect is the relief of hypoxia. Often, the correct diagnosis becomes established during the illness.

Idiopathic Respiratory Distress Syndrome (Hyaline Membrane Disease)

The 1970 UK National Survey of Perinatal Mortality (British Births 1970) showed that idiopathic respiratory distress syndrome (IRDS) was the single most common cause of death in the first week of life, accounting for 3.2 deaths per 1,000 live births and contributing to no less than 30 per cent of all deaths in the first week.

Table 28. Some pulmonary causes of respiratory distress.

A. Common
Idiopathic respiratory distress syndrome
Transient tachypnoea
Pneumothorax
Meconium aspiration syndrome

B. Uncommon
Pneumonia
Pulmonary haemorrhage
Pulmonary hypoplasia
Diaphragmatic hernia
Tracheo-oesophageal fistula
Pulmonary dysfunction of prematurity
(Wilson-Mikity syndrome)

C. Rare
Airway obstruction (choanal atresia, vascular ring, laryngeal web, etc.)
Congenital lobar emphysema
Intrathoracic mass (tumour, cyst, etc.)
Chest wall deformity

Clinical Features

Signs of respiratory distress are present by the time the baby is four hours old. If there has been the opportunity for careful observation from birth, signs are invariably observed in the first hour or two of life. In normal babies, the first 30 minutes or so after birth is a transitional period during which transient and intermittent elevation of the respiratory rate, flaring of the nostrils and minimal chest wall retraction may be observed. In babies with IRDS there is often a prolonged transition which merges imperceptibly with established signs of respiratory distress. IRDS is therefore a disease that truly illustrates the concept of failure of adaptation to extrauterine life.

Generally, the earlier the onset of established signs, the more severe the course of the disease. A carefully observed baby who is free of symptoms at four hours and who later develops respiratory distress is not suffering from IRDS. The disease, if uncomplicated, is self-limiting in that the survivors have clinically recovered by the fourth day.

Diagnosis

The fact that certain antecedent events occur more commonly in babies with IRDS than in normal babies usually provides a pointer to the diagnosis (Table 29). Expiratory grunting and chest-wall retraction are often prominent features (Figure 44). A symmetrical diminution of breath sounds is heard on chest auscultation. However, in the most severe examples of the disease the atelectatic lung may be so solid that it acts as a very efficient conductor of bronchial breath sounds. The chest X-ray appearance is one of diffuse granularity with a superimposed air bronchogram (Figure 45). The granularity is a result of widespread alveolar atelectasis. The bronchial air pattern is readily visualised because it overlies relatively opaque lung fields. An air bronchogram over the cardiac shadow is normal and does not of itself signify IRDS.

Aetiology and Pathogenesis

The most important aetiological factor in IRDS is a deficiency of lung surfactant (Avery and Mead 1959). When air is introduced into the lungs at birth an air/liquid interface forms the lining of the terminal air spaces or alveoli. Stability of the alveolar spaces depends upon the presence at the air/liquid interface of a surface-active material (surfactant) which effectively lowers the surface tension. A relatively high inflationary pressure is required to expand the alveoli of surfactant-deficient lungs, which are described as being 'stiff' or as having a reduced compliance. Less air is retained by the lungs at a given pressure during deflation compared with normal lungs (Figure 46).

A phospholipid, dipalmitoyl lecithin, is the major biochemical component of surfactant in the human lung. Osmiophilic granules seen on microscopy within certain pneumocytes of the alveolar wall probably represent stored surfactant (Figure 47). In fetal life the granules apparently discharge into the fluid-filled alveolar space (Figure 48), and presumably become incorporated into the air/liquid interface.

In babies with IRDS, surfactant regenerates after birth within a few days. However, before this has been completed, a deteriorating cycle of events takes place (Figure 49). Hypoxia and acidaemia in their own right inhibit surfactant production, as does a reduced pulmonary

Table 29. Antecedent events in idiopathic respiratory distress syndrome.

Premature birth
Caesarian section delivery
Ante-partum haemorrhage
Birth asphyxia
Maternal diabetes mellitus
Multiple pregnancy: predilection for the last born

Figure 45. *Chest X-ray in idiopathic respiratory distress syndrome, showing air bronchogram pattern superimposed on relatively opaque lung fields.*

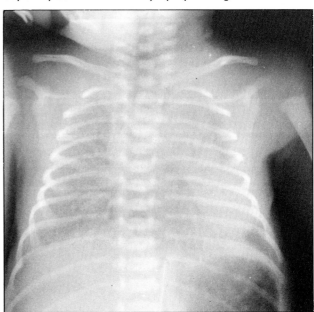

Figure 44. *Chest-wall retraction in a baby with idiopathic respiratory distress syndrome.*

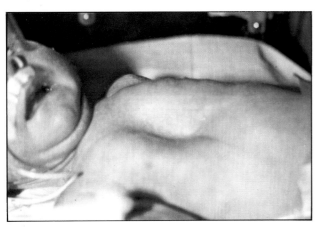

blood flow. In surfactant-deficient lungs the pulmonary capillaries leak plasma into the alveolar space. Fibrin-containing membranes (hyaline membranes) are formed within alveoli (Figure 50). The membranes are not the basic cause of the disease but an associated histological phenomenon.

The most common cause of surfactant deficiency is premature birth. In normal human fetal lung it is not until about 36 weeks that sufficient dipalmitoyl lecithin is present to form a potentially normal air/liquid interface after birth (Gluck *et al.* 1971). However, this does not explain why some very premature babies escape IRDS or why certain term babies suffer from the disease. It seems likely that a surfactant other than dipalmitoyl lecithin is present in fetal lung from as early as 24 weeks' gestation (Gluck *et al.* 1972) and that certain events in fetal life may induce the production of dipalmitoyl lecithin before 36 weeks' gestation (Chiswick 1976). Finally, there are likely to be many factors including hypoxia acting *in utero* or immediately after birth which either inhibit surfactant production or render it inactive.

Treatment

As yet, there is no way of artificially repleting surfactant stores after birth. The management is directed towards providing the best environment that allows the natural replenishment of surfactant, preventing dangerous hypoxia, protecting the baby from the side-effects of treatment and being vigilant for complications associated with the disease. Many aspects of supportive care, particularly with respect to oxygen therapy, are common to other respiratory disorders.

Oxygen administration. Hypoxia plays a key role in the events shown in Figure 49. Prolonged hypoxia is associated with brain damage. Hyperoxaemia in premature babies is associated with retrolental fibroplasia and blindness. A baby who looks pink may be hypoxic or hyperoxaemic. The aim of oxygen therapy is to maintain the partial pressure of oxygen in arterial blood (Po_2) between 50 and 90 mm Hg. Arterial blood may be intermittently sampled (every four to six hours) or continuously analysed from an indwelling umbilical arterial catheter which lies in the abdominal aorta. Alternatively, samples may be intermittently taken from the temporal, brachial or radial arteries. An instrument for measuring blood gases on small quantities of blood (0.4 ml) should be available on all units that undertake the care of babies with IRDS.

Oxygen is a drug. The dose is expressed in percentage

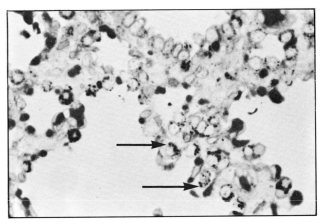

Figure 47. *Light microscopical appearance of pneumocytes which form the walls of the alveolar spaces. Certain pneumocytes contain osmiophilic inclusion granules (arrowed) which are thought to represent stored surfactant ($\times$ 760).*

Figure 46. *Volume-pressure curve of normal lung (A) and surfactant-deficient lung (B). A higher inflationary pressure is required to 'open' B, a smaller volume of air is introduced on inflation to 35 cm H_2O, and on deflation the lungs become virtually airless compared with A.*

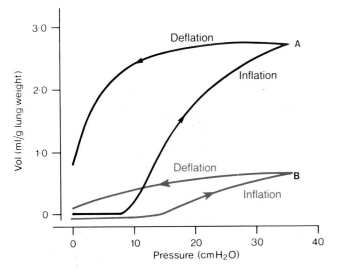

Figure 48. *Electron-microscopical appearance of part of the cell border of a pneumocyte. A vacuole containing osmiophilic material (presumably surfactant) is apparently discharging its contents into the alveolar space. An intact vacuole is also shown ($\times$ 75,000) (Ahmed and Chiswick 1973).*

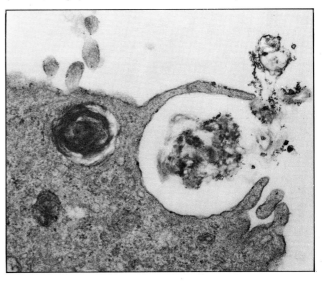

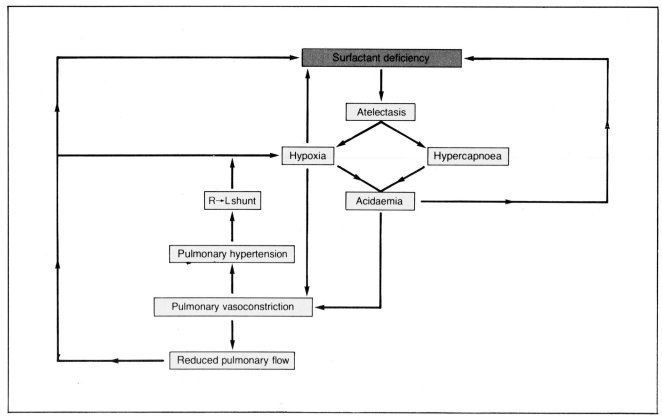

Figure 49. *A vicious cycle of events that is prone to occur in idiopathic respiratory distress syndrome.*

Figure 50. *Lung section from baby who died during idiopathic respiratory distress syndrome. The alveolar space in the centre is completely lined with a pink-staining hyaline membrane, and other alveolar spaces contain membrane remnants (H and E stain).*

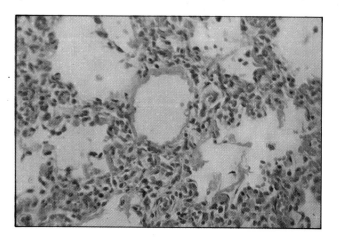

terms and given as continuous therapy. The dose required (ambient oxygen) may be anything from 25 to 100 per cent. The ambient oxygen concentration is measured by an oxygen analyser placed near the baby's mouth. The practice of monitoring oxygen therapy in terms of litres per minute is totally unsatisfactory. This gives no indication of the concentration of oxygen that the baby is breathing. The oxygen should be given into a plastic hood mounted over the baby's head when a concentration of more than 30 per cent is desired (Figure 51). This ensures that the oxygen concentration will not fall significantly should the incubator portholes be opened.

If humidified oxygen is used, care must be taken to avoid the oxygen hood or incubator walls becoming misted, otherwise the baby will be obscured from view, and an environment conducive to the growth of certain 'water bugs', particularly *Pseudomonas*, will be created.

Correction of acidaemia. A mixed respiratory and metabolic acidaemia is commonly present. The blood pH should be maintained above 7.25 by treatment with parenteral sodium bicarbonate. However, a predominantly respiratory acidaemia caused by a raised $P\text{CO}_2$ in arterial blood with a normal and maintained $P\text{O}_2$ will not improve with alkali. When a metabolic component to the acidaemia is suspected, 8.4 per cent sodium bicarbonate should be given in the form of a bolus over 10 to 15 minutes via the umbilical arterial catheter or via a peripheral vein. The suggested dose (Table 30) is designed to undercorrect the acidaemia. The blood pH should be measured 30 minutes later, when a further dose may be given if necessary.

Fluid intake. Most babies will not tolerate oral or nasogastric tube feeds of milk. It is best to provide a peripheral venous infusion of 10 per cent dextrose, starting with 60 ml/kg on the first day and increasing to 120 ml/kg by the third day. By then the baby is usually on the way to recovery and oral or nasogastric tube feeds of milk can be

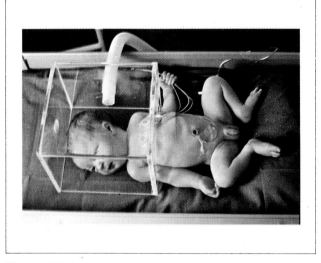

Figure 51. *Perspex hood or head box for the administration of oxygen. An umbilical arterial catheter is in place for the measurement of blood gases. The oxygen analyser for measuring ambient oxygen concentration is not shown, but would normally lie within the head box.*

gradually introduced. It is not generally necessary to add any electrolytes to the dextrose solution.

It is acknowledged that 10 per cent dextrose in the volumes suggested will not fulfil the baby's caloric requirements. The problems and complications associated with maintaining a larger caloric intake during the illness are considerable. Some babies have a severe disease that makes treatment by mechanical ventilation necessary, which in some cases may be prolonged for several weeks. One approach in these circumstances is the feeding of milk through an indwelling nasojejunal tube. In some centres total intravenous nutrition is preferred, in which case fluids, electrolytes, amino acids, lipids, carbohydrate

and vitamins are infused via a catheter sited in a large vein such as the superior vena cava.

The provision of warmth. Subjected to cold stress, the baby needs to increase oxygen consumption and divert calories to maintain a normal rectal temperature. This is undesirable in a baby to whom oxygen and calories are at a premium. Furthermore, hypothermia probably inhibits surfactant production. The baby should be nursed with the chest wall exposed in an incubator which is carefully regulated to maintain the baby within the thermoneutral range. A radiant heat shield reduces radiant heat loss from the baby's skin, but is often an encumbrance to nursing and medical staff. It is too early to assess the efficacy and disadvantages of an alternative approach, which is to nurse the baby outside an incubator exposed to a radiant heat source.

The standard of care a neonatal unit provides for babies with pulmonary problems is measured by the degree of attention to detail the nursing and medical staff display in the provision of basic supportive care as outlined above.

Complications

A common problem is the baby with IRDS who, after an initial improvement, enters a downhill course. Some important causes are shown in Table 31. It must never be assumed that deterioration has occurred because it is inherent in the disease or because an intracranial haemorrhage has occurred. A chest X-ray is mandatory to rule out the possibility of a pneumothorax.

Ventilatory Assistance By Continuous Distending Pressure

An important advance in treatment is the application of a continuous distending pressure to the lungs as the baby breathes spontaneously, which helps the alveoli to remain open during expiration. A dramatic reduction in the oxygen requirement is often seen in babies who before

Table 30. Dose of intravenous sodium bicarbonate (8.4 per cent) for the treatment of acidaemia in IRDS.

Blood pH	Dose (ml/kg body weight)
< 7.0	7.0
7.0 – 7.09	5.0
7.1 – 7.19	4.0
7.2 – 7.24	3.0

Table 31. Causes of deterioration in idiopathic respiratory distress syndrome.

Pneumothorax
Pneumonia
Pulmonary haemorrhage
Intraventricular haemorrhage
Peripheral circulatory failure
Hypoglycaemia

Figure 52. *Baby with idiopathic respiratory distress syndrome receiving continuous positive airways pressure treatment within a Gregory box. A sleeve of polythene acts as the neck seal.*

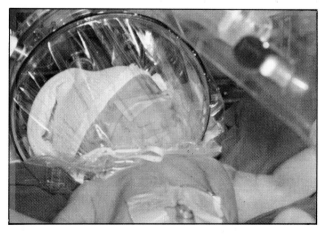

treatment required an oxygen concentration of 60 per cent or more to achieve a normal Po_2.

The continuous distending pressure is achieved by the application to the airway of a positive pressure of up to 10 cm H_2O. Several methods exist:

1. Head box (Gregory box). The baby's head is placed in a perspex box or cylinder. A sleeve of polythene serves as a neck seal (Figure 52). The mean positive pressure inside the box is regulated by the flow rate of oxygen or air/oxygen mixture into the box and by a variable blow-off valve incorporated into the wall of the box.

2. Endotracheal tube.

3. Face mask.

4. Nasal prongs.

The circuit used for applying CPAP by methods 2, 3 or 4 is similar and is shown in Figure 53.

Continuous negative pressure to chest wall (CNP): the thorax of the baby is sealed in a perspex chamber at a constant negative pressure of up to 10 cm H_2O. The resultant negative intrapleural pressure subjects the airways to a continuous distending pressure.

All methods of applying a continuous distending pressure carry the risk of pneumothorax. Each method has its special merits and side-effects.

Figure 53. *Diagram of circuit for administering continuous positive airways pressure (CPAP) treatment by methods other than a Gregory box.*
A To patient via endotracheal tube, nasal prongs or face mask
B Flow of humidified oxygen or air/oxygen mixture
C Pressure gauge
D T-piece
E Corrugated tubing
F Water manometer serving as a blow-off safety valve
G Anaesthetic bag (500 ml)
H Screw clamp which regulates the pressure within the circuit by adjusting the degree of leak at the end of the anaesthetic bag.

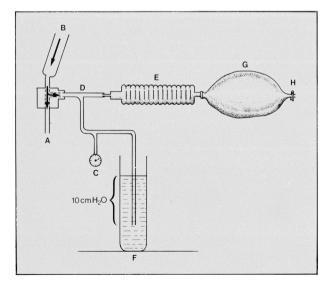

Table 32. Indications for mechanical ventilation in idiopathic respiratory distress syndrome.

Recurrent apnoeic episodes or a single major apnoeic attack.
Arterial Po_2 < 40 mm Hg in an ambient oxygen concentration of 95–100 per cent.
Arterial Pco_2 > 90 mm Hg associated with a pH < 7.2 in spite of alkali treatment.

Ventilatory Assistance by Mechanical Ventilation

The indications for mechanical ventilation are shown in Table 32. It is stressed that this method of treatment should only be performed in units especially staffed and equipped for this purpose. An adult intensive care unit is certainly not the place for such babies to be nursed, nor is it generally desirable for newborn babies to be nursed in a children's intensive care unit. Ventilatory support is only one aspect of treatment of the ill neonate with IRDS. Optimal care is best achieved when the baby is looked after in a neonatal intensive care unit under the supervision of a neonatologist who is committed to this speciality.

Results of Treatment

Survival rates of about 70 per cent for very ill babies with IRDS requiring mechanical ventilation are now being reported by some centres. It is particularly encouraging that neurological sequelae are no more frequent in premature babies who have survived IRDS than in babies of an equivalent gestational age who have escaped this disease (Robertson and Crichton 1969). More important than neurological sequelae in survivors is the development of chronic pulmonary insufficiency (bronchopulmonary dysplasia) in certain babies who have required mechanical ventilation with high concentrations of oxygen for longer than five to six days.

Transient Tachypnoea of the Newborn

This descriptive term is applicable to certain neonates who develop signs of respiratory distress immediately after birth. Tachypnoea is the prominent physical sign with perhaps minimal chest wall retraction on inspiration. Babies of any gestational age may be affected, although it is more common in those born at term. Personal experience suggests that birth by elective caesarean section is a predisposing factor. Babies rarely require more than 30 per cent oxygen to achieve a satisfactory arterial Po_2, and acidaemia and hypercapnoea are not present. The elevation of the respiratory rate may persist for up to five days and complications have not been reported.

One suggestion is that a delay in the clearance of fetal lung fluid is responsible for the syndrome. In keeping with this the chest X-ray has an ill-defined streaky appearance radiating from the hila (Figure 54) or prominent reticular shadows which suggest the presence of dilated lymphatics. Small pleural effusions in the costophrenic angles and interlobar fissures are common.

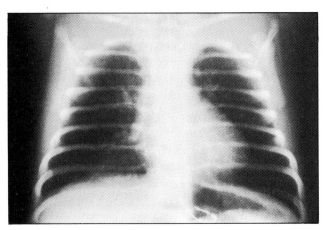

Figure 54. *Transient tachypnoea. There are prominent vascular markings radiating from the hila.*

Figure 55. *There is a pneumothorax on the left side. A pleural drain is* in situ. *Interstitial emphysema is particularly well shown in the right lung by the appearance of irregular translucencies.*

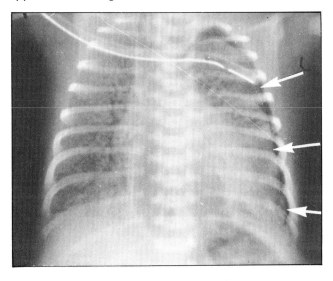

Table 33. Situations in which a pneumothorax is prone to occur.

Positive pressure ventilation during resuscitation at birth.
Assisted ventilation treatment for pulmonary disease:
a) Positive pressure ventilation.
b) Continuous positive airways pressure.
c) Continuous negative pressure to chest wall.
Meconium aspiration syndrome.
Idiopathic respiratory distress syndrome.
Hypoplastic lungs in association with Potter's syndrome.
Diaphragmatic hernia.
Obstructive urological malformations.

Figure 56. *Lateral decubitus view, left side raised, demonstrates a left pneumothorax which was not visible on an A-P view. Arrows indicate the margin of the left lung and the gas bubble in the stomach.*

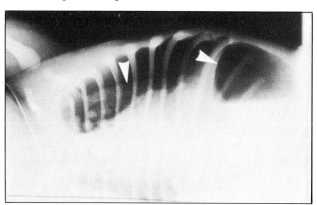

Pneumothorax

Alveolar rupture is usually associated with dissection of air along vascular sheaths (interstitial emphysema, see Figure 55) and the subsequent accumulation of air in the mediastinal space (pneumomediastinum), as well as in the pleural cavity (pneumothorax, see Figure 55). The first breath is associated with the transient occurrence of an intrathoracic pressure sometimes approaching 100 cm H_2O. This may explain why an asymptomatic pneumothorax, detected by chest X-ray, is present in one to two per cent of all newborn babies. Other situations in which a pneumothorax is prone to occur are shown in Table 33.

The clinical signs are those of respiratory distress, with tachypnoea being prominent. Although displacement of the apex beat is a helpful sign, a normally positioned apex beat does not exclude the diagnosis. Whereas diminished breath sounds and a hyper-resonant percussion note on the affected side are frequently heard in an adult, they

are often not detected in the neonate. A chest X-ray is required for diagnosis, and radiographic examination should be made on all babies with respiratory distress. It must be stressed that routine A-P views often fail to reveal the true extent of a pneumothorax and on occasion may appear normal in an affected baby. When a pneumothorax is clinically suspected or when a baby has respiratory distress and an apparently normal A-P chest X-ray, lateral decubitus views with right and left sides up should be obtained. This allows a collection of pleural air, previously undetected, to become visible (Figure 56).

The treatment is dictated by clinical circumstances. When a pneumothorax is suspected in a baby whose state is rapidly deteriorating, temporary drainage of the pleural cavity should be carried out immediately. A bevelled needle (No. 18) attached via a three-way tap to a syringe (20 ml) is inserted to a depth of 1 to 1.5 cm in the second intercostal space at the mid-clavicular line on the suspected side. When a tension pneumothorax is present there is usually no difficulty in aspirating air. If air cannot be aspirated there should be no hesitation in repeating the procedure on the contralateral side. The neonate's powers of deception with respect to physical signs are quite remarkable!

Formal underwater drainage of a pneumothorax should normally be performed in a baby with respiratory symptoms after the lesion has been diagnosed by chest X-ray. A cannula is inserted on a trochar into the pleural cavity at the site recommended above, and connected to an underwater drainage bottle. Unless a large enough cannula is used (10 or 12 French gauge) it will readily become blocked. If there is delay or difficulty in establishing formal drainage, the administration of 100 per cent oxygen by face mask accelerates the absorption of air in the pleural cavity. Nitrogen is 'washed out' of the blood, thereby creating a difference in the total gas tension between the gas in the pleural space and that in the blood. If this method is used, frequent clinical observations are necessary and a needle, three-way tap and syringe should be available for emergency use.

Meconium Aspiration Syndrome

The passage of meconium into the amniotic fluid and gasping *in utero* are features of fetal asphyxia. Inhalation of meconium results in the development of a chemical pneumonitis and plugging of the airways. The meconium plugs may act as ball-valve obstructions and so contribute to the overall pulmonary pathology, which consists of areas of consolidation or under-aeration and areas of hyperinflation.

The characteristic presentation is of irregular gasping respiration at birth in a meconium-stained baby. Laryngoscopy and removal by suction of any obstructing meconium should be rapidly performed before starting positive pressure ventilation. It is desirable to aspirate the stomach to avoid the risk of further meconium inhalation should the baby vomit. Signs of respiratory distress develop soon after resuscitation. Tachypnoea is the prominent feature and, in contrast to the premature baby with IRDS, the chest often appears enlarged because of air trapping. The chest X-ray shows coarse widely scattered densities (Figure 57). Pneumomediastinum and pneumothorax are important complications that occur

Figure 57. *Meconium aspiration syndrome. There is increased opacity of both lungs, and coarse ill-defined mottling is seen in the right lower zone.*

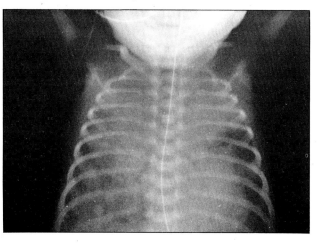

Table 34. Factors that suggest the diagnosis of pneumonia in the newborn with respiratory distress.

Suggestive chest X-ray appearance.

Neutrophil polymorph count $> 7,000/mm^3$ after the fourth day, or $< 1,500/mm^3$ at any time.

Suspicious antecedent events:
a) Prolonged rupture of membranes (> 24 hours).
b) Maternal fever within a few days before birth.
c) Abnormal maternal vaginal discharge.
d) Foul-smelling liquor amnii.
e) Premature birth.

Unexpected deterioration during the course of pre-existing lung disease, particularly IRDS and meconium aspiration syndrome.

Confirmed sepsis at other sites, e.g. septicaemia, meningitis.

Exposure to ventilatory apparatus.

in ten to 20 per cent of cases, and may even be noted on the initial X-ray.

The basis of treatment is the provision of humidified oxygen at a concentration that achieves a satisfactory arterial Po_2, the correction of acidaemia and basic supportive care. Antibiotics (e.g. penicillin and gentamicin) should be given because it is not possible radiologically or clinically to distinguish pneumonia from meconium aspiration. Furthermore, intratracheal meconium in rats was shown to enhance susceptibility to *E. coli* infection (Bryan 1967). It is prudent to perform 12-hourly chest X-rays in the seriously ill neonate because the clinical signs of a pneumothorax may not readily be detected.

Those babies who recover usually do so in 48 hours, although persistent tachypnoea and delayed radiological clearing for one to two weeks is occasionally observed. In contrast to IRDS, survival rates are very low in neonates who require mechanical ventilation for respiratory distress caused by meconium aspiration.

Pneumonia

Pneumonia is now an uncommon cause of death in the newborn period, contributing to one per cent of all deaths in the first week of life (British Births 1970). The reported incidence of the disease varies considerably in different centres and obviously depends on the diagnostic criteria used (Table 34). Pneumonia is distinctly uncommon as a cause of respiratory distress on the author's unit, and is almost confined to neonates who have acquired the disease as a complication of some form of assisted ventilation treatment.

Congenital pneumonia is usually the result of organisms penetrating the uterine cavity from the birth canal, and the clinical signs are present at or soon after birth. The organisms most commonly cultured from amniotic fluid or from the baby's lungs at postmortem are *E. coli*, streptococci and staphylococci. In contrast, *Pseudomonas* is a well-recognised cause of postnatally acquired pneumonia in those babies receiving assisted ventilation treatment and exposed to warm moist apparatus.

A high index of suspicion is necessary for the recognition of the disease, with special attention to the events preceding the onset of signs (Table 34). The non-specific signs of sepsis often overshadow those of respiratory distress. Auscultatory signs of lobar distribution are rarely elicited and indeed the breath sounds are often normal. The chest X-ray is the most helpful diagnostic aid. The appearance is of bilateral or unilateral coarse, ill-defined mottling (Figure 58). Attention has previously been drawn to the difficulty in distinguishing pneumonia from the meconium aspiration syndrome on clinical and radiological grounds.

Treatment is directed towards the prevention of hypoxia and acidaemia, the provision of basic supportive care, and the eradication of the infecting organism by the use of antibiotics. Occasionally, in congenital infection there is a clue to the causative organism from the results of amniotic fluid, placental or vaginal swab culture. Culture of the pharyngeal aspirate is generally unhelpful because the organisms grown do not necessarily reflect the organisms in the lung. A combination of antibiotics active against a broad spectrum of organisms should be used (e.g. penicillin and gentamicin) and these may have to be changed in the light of the baby's progress

Pulmonary Hypoplasia

Hypoplastic lungs are usually associated with other congenital malformations, particularly diaphragmatic hernia (Figure 60). Another malformation frequently associated with pulmonary hypoplasia is renal agenesis (Potter 1946). In this condition (Potter's syndrome) there is a

Figure 58. *Mottling is seen throughout the lung fields in this neonate who developed* Pseudomonas *pneumonia during assisted ventilation treatment for IRDS. The opacities are much more coarse than the granular opacities seen in uncomplicated IRDS, although the appearances would also be compatible with meconium aspiration syndrome.*

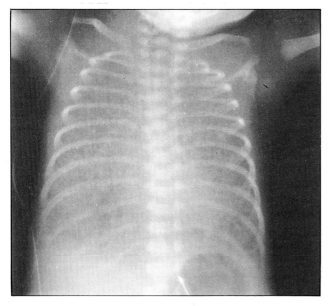

characteristic facial appearance with low-set ears, prominent epicanthic folds, flattened nose and a small chin (Figure 59), and invariably a history of oligohydramnios.

Severe pulmonary hypoplasia is associated with death soon after birth because the lungs cannot be readily inflated when resuscitation is attempted. Babies with less severe pulmonary hypoplasia may survive for a varying length of time after birth and have signs of respiratory distress. Cyanosis is a prominent feature and may be caused by right to left shunting of blood through the hypoplastic lungs or by the associated presence of congenital heart disease or both. Occasionally the pulmonary lesion is amenable to surgical treatment by resection of one vestigial lung.

Apnoeic Attacks and Periodic Breathing

About 30 to 50 per cent of premature babies have spells of periodic breathing consisting of brief pauses in ventilation of about five to ten seconds duration, alternating with periods of ventilation at a rate of about 50 to 60 per minute. It is more commonly observed after the first few days of life and may persist for six weeks. In contrast to prolonged apnoeic episodes (see below), bradycardia is not a feature, and the pH of 'arterialised' capillary blood is usually slightly alkalotic, e.g. 7.44. The precise aetiology is unknown (Hornbein 1972). Although periodic breathing is common in premature babies it cannot be assumed that this pattern of breathing is entirely harmless. We are once again reminded that normality of a particular condition cannot be assumed merely because it is frequently observed in premature babies. Prematurity itself is a pathological entity.

About 30 per cent of premature babies who weigh less than 1,750 g at birth have prolonged apnoeic attacks of more than 15 seconds duration. These spells are usually limited to the first two weeks of life and when prolonged may be associated with bradycardia, cyanosis, and metabolic acidosis. Many diverse neonatal conditions may be heralded by apnoeic episodes. The diagnostic label of 'apnoea of prematurity' must not be used without a consideration of the differential diagnosis (Table 35). However, in many cases there is no satisfactory explanation for these episodes, which are often attributed to the presence of an 'immature respiratory centre'. The fact that most affected babies apparently breathe normally for several days before the onset of apnoeic attacks makes this concept rather naïve.

Treatment of Apnoeic Attacks

The prime aim is the prevention of dangerous hypoxaemia. If an apnoeic episode is detected early, simple methods of stimulating the baby usually readily provoke the onset of breathing. Intermittent nursing observations are certainly not sufficient for the early recognition of apnoea. There are many different types of respiration-dependent apnoea monitors available, which alarm during an apnoeic spell after a variable preset delay (5 to 15 seconds). One problem with respiration-dependent

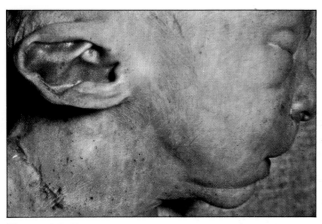

Figure 59. *The facial appearance in Potter's syndrome. Note the low-set malformed ears, flattened nose, and small chin. Prominent epicanthic folds were also present.*

monitors is their tendency to give false alarms, particularly in very low birthweight babies. An alternative or additional approach is to monitor the heart rate, which becomes slower in association with apnoea. Some argue that the presence of bradycardia does not consistently provide an early enough warning of significant apnoea. All babies less than 34 weeks gestation should be monitored for apnoeic attacks during the first two weeks of life. If an attack does not promptly respond to cutaneous stimulation, the baby should be ventilated with air or 30 per cent oxygen using a bag and mask until spontaneous respiration is resumed, which is often within a minute or two. It is unnecessary to ventilate with higher concentrations of oxygen except in the presence of an underlying lung disease (e.g. IRDS) that necessitated oxygen therapy before the occurrence of apnoea.

Prophylaxis of Apnoeic Attacks

Servo-controlling the environmental temperature to achieve a skin temperature of less than 1°C below normal significantly reduced the number of apnoeic episodes in a group of premature babies (Dailey *et al.* 1969). This at least suggests that babies with apnoeic episodes should be nursed at the lower end of the thermoneutral range.

A decrease in the frequency of apnoeic attacks is sometimes observed if the ambient oxygen concentration is in-

Table 35. Certain neonatal conditions that may present with apnoeic episodes.

Sepsis.
Hypoglycaemia.
Electrolyte disturbances.
Drug depression as a result of the transplacental passage of analgesic agents used in labour.
Intracranial haemorrhage.
Manifestations of convulsions.

creased to 25 to 30 per cent. It may be criminally negligent to nurse a premature baby with apnoeic attacks in 'just a whiff of oxygen' without measuring the ambient oxygen concentrations. The risk of retrolental fibroplasia is of course related to the arterial P_{O_2}. A premature baby with 'normal' lungs can certainly develop the disease by breathing more than 40 per cent oxygen for several hours. The use of 25 to 30 per cent oxygen for the prophylaxis of apnoeic attacks is only justified if an accurate oxygen analyser is used and the nursing and medical staff are vigilant.

The use of aminophylline (Kuzemko and Paala 1973), theophylline or caffeine benzoate often reduces the frequency of apnoeic attacks, although their mechanism of action is unknown. As an example, 2 to 3 mg/kg of theophylline may be given orally every six hours to maintain blood levels of 6 to 12 μg /ml.

The use of continuous positive airways pressure is sometimes associated with a reduction in the frequency of apnoeic episodes, although the mechanism is imperfectly understood. Any beneficial effect has to be weighed against the known side-effects of CPAP. A head box device for giving CPAP should certainly not be used under these circumstances because the baby is not readily accessible should a major apnoeic episode occur. The use of CPAP via an indwelling endotracheal tube, nasal prongs or an attached face mask has the bonus that the baby can be readily hand ventilated for brief periods if necessary.

Mechanical ventilation is used for babies having prolonged and/or very frequent apnoeic attacks associated with cyanosis and metabolic acidosis.

Some Surgical Conditions Associated with Respiratory Distress

Respiratory distress may be caused by a congenital malformation amenable to surgical treatment. Affected babies are often born in a hospital where no team of neonatal surgeons and anaesthetists is immediately available. It is necessary for all those caring for the newborn to be able to provide effective 'first aid' treatment, pending advice from surgeon and anaesthetist colleagues. Details of transportation of such babies to a neonatal surgical centre are beyond the scope of this discussion. Three surgical conditions that have immediate therapeutic implications will be considered.

Diaphragmatic Hernia

Usually herniation of the abdominal viscera into the thoracic cavity occurs through the foramen of Bochdalek on the left side. The severity of symptoms depends on the volume of abdominal viscera within the chest (Figure 60). Many affected babies fail to establish respiration after birth and rapidly deteriorate in spite of expert care. In others respiration is established with difficulty, and signs of respiratory distress, particularly cyanosis, are present from birth. Clues to the diagnosis are presented in Table 36. However, it should be stressed that none of these signs

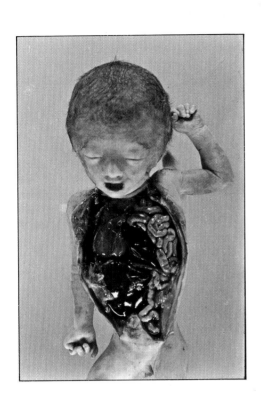

Figure 60. *Diaphragmatic hernia in a neonate who also had hypoplastic lungs in association with Potter's syndrome. A portion of liver and a considerable length of bowel have herniated through the left side of the diaphragm into the thoracic cavity. The heart is displaced to the right. Some of the facial characteristics of Potter's syndrome are also shown.*

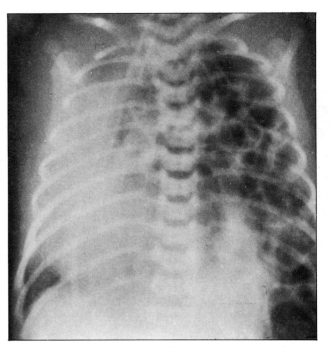

Figure 61. *Left-sided diaphragmatic hernia. The translucencies in the left hemithorax are loops of bowel containing air. The cardiac shadow occupies most of the right hemithorax. The endotracheal tube, through which the baby was being ventilated, is displaced to the right, an illustration of the mediastinal displacement. This baby was operated on, and is now one year old and thriving normally.*

is invariably present. The diagnosis is confirmed by chest X-ray (Figure 61).

Operative mortality is powerfully influenced by the promptness of referral to a neonatal surgical unit and the standard of pre-operative care. The following are some important guides to pre-operative management:

1. Aspirate the stomach via a nasogastric tube continuously or at intervals of five minutes.

2. Give positive pressure ventilation via an endotracheal tube with sufficient concentration of oxygen to alleviate cyanosis. Ventilatory pressures should normally not exceed 20 cm H_2O, and because of the real risk of the development of a tension pneumothorax, a needle, three-way tap and syringe should be readily available (see treatment of pneumothorax, pages 53 to 54).

3. Nurse the baby on the side of the hernia with the head of the cot or incubator slightly raised.

Tracheo-Oesophageal Fistula

Most cases are associated with oesophageal atresia with the fistulous connection between the trachea and distal segment of the atretic oesophagus. Associated anomalies, particularly anorectal malformations, are present in about 50 per cent of affected babies.

Characteristically, frothy saliva is seen flowing from the mouth. This is associated with episodic choking and respiratory distress, cyanosis being a prominent feature. If the baby is fed, the symptoms become worse and aspiration pneumonitis and pulmonary collapse may ensue. A history of hydramnios should alert the attendant to the diagnosis, which may be confirmed by passing a radio-opaque catheter (No. 10 French gauge) into the oesophagus via a nostril. In the presence of oesophageal atresia the catheter cannot be advanced into the stomach and the site of obstruction is confirmed by chest and abdominal X-ray.

An important feature of pre-operative management is the need to keep the upper oesophageal segment empty of saliva by gentle intermittent aspiration via a naso-oesophageal tube. The frequency of aspiration is governed

Table 36. Physical signs that may be present in the newborn with diaphragmatic hernia.

1. Apex beat displaced to opposite side.
2. On the side of the lesion:
   a) Diminished chest wall movements.
   b) Diminished breath sounds.
   c) Bowel sounds present.
3. Scaphoid abdomen.

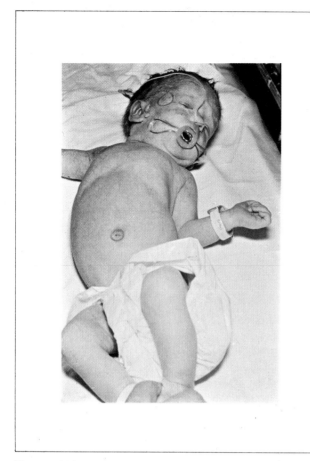

Figure 62. *This neonate has complete choanal atresia on the left side, and severe choanal narrowing on the right. Respiratory distress was present at rest. Pre-operatively the baby was fed via a nasogastric tube on the right side which was passed with difficulty beyond the nasopharynx. An oral airway is in situ, and in spite of this some subcostal recession is still present.*

by the rate at which secretions accumulate. Freeman (1969) recommends that the baby should be nursed on alternate sides every one to two hours, presumably to encourage pulmonary drainage and prevent lung collapse. The upper oesophageal pouch should be suctioned immediately before the baby's position is changed. Some think it desirable to maintain an atmosphere of high humidity which may reduce the tenacity of the sputum.

Choanal Atresia

About two-thirds of reported cases are unilateral and are usually not recognised in the neonatal period. In bilateral choanal atresia respiratory distress is usually present from birth. Prominent features are cyanosis, thoracic cage retraction, and indrawing of the lips and cheeks on inspiration. The symptoms are rapidly relieved when the baby cries or when an oral airway is inserted. In some babies the symptoms are episodic and are particularly associated with feeding. The diagnosis is suggested by the lack of free passage of a soft rubber catheter through the nostrils past the pharynx.

Respiratory distress should be promptly relieved by insertion of an oral airway, pending surgical treatment (Figure 62). Feeding can be achieved via an indwelling orogastric tube adjacent to the airway, or by spoon with temporary removal of the oral airway.

References

Ahmed, A. and Chiswick, M. L., *J. Path.,* 1974, **113,** 161.

Avery, M. E. and Mead, J., *Am. J. Dis. Child.,* 1959, **97,** 517.

British Births 1970, Vol. 1, *The First Week of Life,* Heinemann Medical Books Ltd., London, 1975.

Bryan, C. S., *Johns Hopkins Med. J.,* 1967, **121,** 9.

Chiswick, M. L., *Arch. Dis. Childh.,* 1976, **51,** 674.

Dailey, W., Klaus, M. and Meyer, H., *Pediatrics,* 1969, **43,** 510.

Freeman, N. V., in *Neonatal Surgery,* (page 207), (eds. Rickham, P. P. and Johnston, J. H.), Butterworth, London, 1969.

Gluck, L., Kulovich, M. V., Borer, R. C., Brenner, P. H., Anderson, C. G. and Spellacy, W. N., *Amer. J. Obstet. Gynec.,* 1971, **109,** 440.

Gluck, L., Kulovich, M. V., Eidelman, A. I., Cordero, L. and Khazin, A. F., *Pediat. Res.,* 1972, **6,** 81.

Hornbein, T. F., *Pediatrics,* 1972, **50,** 183.

Kuzemko, J. A. and Paala, J., *Arch. Dis. Child.,* 1973, **48,** 404.

Potter, E. L., *J. Pediat.,* 1946, **29,** 68.

Robertson, A. M. and Crichton, J. U., *Amer. J. Dis. Child.,* 1969, **117,** 271.

Further Reading

Avery, M. E. and Fletcher, B. D., *The Lung and its Disorders in the Newborn Infant,* W. B. Saunders, Philadelphia, 1974.

Chernick, V. (Ed.), Onset and control of fetal and neonatal respiration, in *Seminars in Perinatology,* 1977, **1,** Grune and Stratton, New York.

9. Neurological Problems

Neonates with neurological problems may present in three ways:

1. Abnormal neurological behaviour patterns.
2. Congenital malformations of the central nervous system.
3. Traumatic nerve palsies.

Abnormal Neurological Behaviour

The neonate reacts in a limited and stereotyped way to diverse neurological disorders. Numerous conditions other than primary abnormalities of the nervous system present with neurological manifestations. The common abnormal behaviour patterns are shown in Table 37. Several types of abnormal behaviour usually occur together. Apathy may be associated with a weak cry, respiratory depression and floppiness. Hyperexcitability may occur with jitteriness, fits, hypertonia and a shrill cry. Occasionally one particular feature dominates the picture, e.g. fits or floppiness. The problem is that no single aspect or combination of abnormal behaviour is one characteristic of a pathological lesion (Table 38).

Clinical Diagnosis

The diagnostic approach in the neonate is somewhat different from the traditional method used in adult neurology, where the mode of presentation and the nature of the symptoms often give clues to the pathology of the lesion. In the neonate, knowledge of the events and circumstances before and following birth is more likely to be informative (Figure 63). Neurological examination in the adult may clearly point to the site of the lesion. This is rarely so in the neonate presenting with an abnormal behaviour pattern, where at best the examination may reveal abnormal signs supporting the presence of abnormal behaviour, and may, when floppiness is the main feature, distinguish 'cerebral' disturbances from the rarer neuromuscular or muscular abnormalities.

Neurological Examination

This is an extension of the general examination, with particular focus on the nervous system. There are certain pitfalls.

1. The neonate's state of wakefulness (Prechtl and Beintema 1964) powerfully influences the findings. It is best to examine when the baby is awake with eyes open, but not incessantly crying. When repeated observations at different times suggest that this state cannot be achieved, this may in itself be an important finding.

2. Posture, muscle tone, spontaneous movements and the presence of primitive neonatal reflexes are influenced by gestational age.

3. When assessing muscle tone and tendon jerks, ensure that the baby's head is held in the midline, otherwise spurious results are obtained.

4. Do not be obsessed with repeatedly trying to elicit a physical sign because of uncertainty of its presence. Instead, acknowledge the uncertainty, document it and leave it at that, because an acknowledged uncertainty is more informative than a false result.

5. Examination performed immediately after a fit is generally unhelpful.

General Observations

Observe the posture, spontaneous movements and respiratory activity. A persistent wide-awake, staring appearance is a feature of a cerebral disturbance and may be seen in hyperexcitable or otherwise apathetic neonates (Figure 64). Valuable information about muscle tone may be obtained when undressing the baby. Hypotonic neonates generally part with their clothes readily.

Head and Spine

1. Measure the occipitofrontal head circumference (OFC) and plot it on a centile chart which relates OFC to conceptional age.

2. Assess the tension of the anterior fontanelle.

Table 37. Abnormal neurological behaviour patterns.

Apathy, paucity of movement
Floppiness
Hyperexcitability
Convulsions, jitteriness
Impaired sucking and swallowing
Shallow, irregular respiration or apnoeic attacks
Absent, weak or shrill cry

Hypoxia	Birth trauma	Drugs	Sepsis

Growth-retarded fetus
Prolonged labour
Meconium stained liquor
Abnormal fetal heart rate
Fetal acidosis
Delayed onset of
  respiration
	Small for dates
	Large for dates
	Abnormal presenting part
	Manipulative delivery
	Bruised baby
		Dose and time of drugs
		given during labour and
		delivery, including local
		anaesthetics
		Drug addiction:
		  history of jaundice
		  infected venepuncture
		   sites
		  occupations at risk
			Transplacental:
			  illness in pregnancy
			  known contact
			Abnormal vaginal
			  discharge
			Maternal fever
			Purulent liquor
			Prematurity
			Contact with warm,
			  moist apparatus

Non-traumatic intracranial haemorrhage	Metabolic	Neuromuscular

Bleeding from other sites
Prematurity
Idiopathic respiratory
 distress
Apnoeic attacks
	Hypoglycaemia:
	  small for dates
	  hypoxic insult
	  diabetic mother
	  exchange transfusion
	Inborn error:
	  family history
	  urine smell
	  unexplained acidosis
	  unexplained alkalosis
	  onset when reasonable
	  milk intake achieved
		Family history
		Poor fetal movements
		Maternal myasthenia
		  or myotonia

Figure 63. *Clues to be sought in the diagnosis of abnormal neurological behaviour.*

3. Examine the skull sutures; remember that widely separated sutures do not indicate hydrocephalus unless the OFC is abnormally large.

4. Observe the facial appearance. Abnormal neurological behaviour in association with an unusual facial appearance might suggest a chromosomal abnormality. Down's syndrome is by far the most common example (associated with floppiness).

5. Examine for midline spinal abnormalities.

Retinoscopy

This is generally uninformative, and there is little point in struggling for a long time with a baby merely to catch a fleeting glimpse of the retina. Retinal haemorrhages are seen in apparently normal babies (Baum and Bulpitt 1970), and papilloedema is not a feature of raised intracranial pressure in the newborn.

Cranial Nerves

The traditional examination of each cranial nerve as performed in adult neurology is rarely helpful in the neonate, unless a specific cranial nerve abnormality is suspected (e.g. ptosis or bilateral facial palsy). Eye movements may be assessed by gently rotating the baby's head from side to side; normally, the eyes should keep a constant position in space. The pupillary reaction to light, which appears at 29 to 31 weeks gestation (Robinson 1966), may be absent when intracranial pressure is raised. The optic pathways deserve special mention in that the ability of the neonate to fixate and follow a moving object (e.g. small red ball held 30 cm from the eyes) is probably a useful index of cortical function. Certain neonatal reflexes have cranial nerve pathways (e.g. sucking, rooting, glabellar tap) but failure to elicit a response in a mature baby usually indicates 'cerebral depression' rather than a cranial nerve abnormality.

Spontaneous Movements

These should be assessed at intervals throughout the examination, remembering that the degree of spontaneous movement is influenced by the baby's 'state' and maturity. The consistent finding of a paucity of movement is as important as the occurrence of abnormal movements, e.g. jitteriness or fits. Observe for asymmetry of movement.

Posture and Muscle Tone

Posture is an important indication of the distribution and degree of muscle tone. The baby should be observed in the prone and supine position on a flat surface (Figure 65), and held by the examiner with one hand supporting the baby's trunk. When assessing resistance to passive movements of the limbs, importance should only be attached to gross abnormalities of tone or definite asymmetry. The abdomen of a baby with significant hypotonia is remarkably easy to examine, the abdominal musculature offering little resistance.

Table 38. Causes of abnormal neurological behaviour.

1. Hypoxia
   antepartum
   intrapartum
   neonatal

2. Birth trauma
   torn dural sinus
   ruptured great cerebral vein
   subdural haemorrhage
   injury to cervical cord

3. Maternal drugs
   analgesics/sedatives in labour
   local anaesthetics
   drug addiction

4. Sepsis
   antepartum
   intrapartum
   neonatal

5. Electrolyte disturbance
   hypocalcaemia
   hypomagnesaemia
   hypernatraemia
   hyponatraemia

6. Metabolic disturbance
   inborn error of protein metabolism
   pyridoxine dependency
   galactosaemia
   hyperbilirubinaemia
   hypoglycaemia
   hypothyroidism
   hyperthyroidism

7. Non-traumatic intracranial haemorrhage
   intraventricular
   subarachnoid

8. Structural cerebral abnormality
   hydrocephalus
   microcephaly
   porencephalic cyst
   hydranencephaly
   encephalocele
   subarachnoid cyst

9. Neuromuscular abnormality
   spinal muscular atrophy (Werdnig–Hoffmann)
   transient myasthenia gravis
   congenital myopathy
   glycogen storage disease of muscle
   dystrophia myotonica

10. Chromosome abnormality
    Down's syndrome (trisomy 21)
    Edward's syndrome (trisomy 18)
    Patau syndrome (trisomy 13, 15)
    cri-du-chat syndrome

Tendon Reflexes

The ease of elicitation of tendon reflexes varies widely in normal neonates and very brisk responses are often observed. Although normal responses may be obtained in neonates with muscle disorders, the presence of normal tendon reflexes in the lower limbs of a floppy baby makes the diagnosis of spinal muscular atrophy most unlikely. The examination may also be helpful in providing supportive evidence of asymmetrical neurological signs and in the assessment of the level of a myelomeningocele.

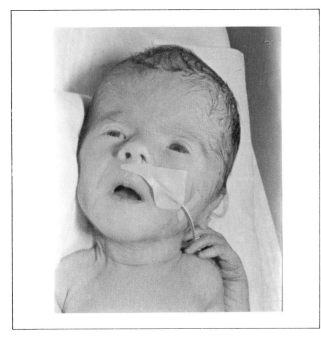

Figure 64. *This small for dates, premature neonate suffered from severe intrapartum hypoxia. The persistent staring appearance of the eyes contrasted with his apathetic, hypotonic behaviour.*

Primitive Neonatal Reflexes

There are numerous primitive neonatal reflexes, and impaired or exaggerated responses are observed with 'cerebral depression' (apathy) and hyperexcitability respectively. Certain reflexes have already been discussed in Chapter 4. Others are described below.

1. *Moro's reflex.* The baby is held in the supine position, with the head cradled in the examiner's left hand and the trunk supported by the right arm and hand. When the head is suddenly allowed to fall a few centimetres, abduction and extension of the upper limbs is immediately followed by adduction and flexion.

2. *Sucking reflex.* Observe for sucking movements in response to a clean finger placed in the baby's mouth.

3. *Palmar grasp reflex.* The handle of a small tendon hammer is placed across the palmar surface of the baby's fingers. Flexion of the digits is promptly seen.

4. *Babkin's sign.* The examiner's thumbs are pressed firmly but gently into the baby's palms, with the baby's hands loosely held. The mouth promptly opens and the tongue protrudes. The test is less unpleasant for the baby than the elicitation of Moro's reflex, and in the author's experience consistent failure to elicit a response is a useful index of 'cerebral depression'.

Elicitation of Babinski's Sign

This is an important part of the examination in the adult. However, different observers rarely agree on its presence or absence in an individual neonate or on its significance. It is probably best omitted when time is at a premium.

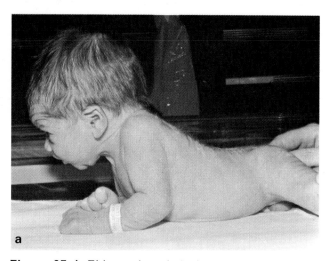

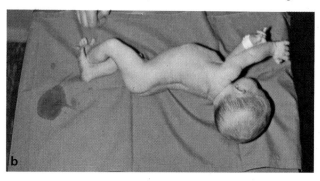

Figure 65a). *This newborn baby has extensor hypertonus probably resulting from intrapartum hypoxia, and shows the false appearance of being developmentally advanced.* **b)** *Gross extensor hypertonus (opisthotonus) in a neonate with meningitis.*

Sensation

Generally no useful purpose is served in subjecting the baby to unpleasant pinpricks, and this test should be omitted except when assessing the level of a myelomeningocele.

Causes of Abnormal Neurological Behaviour

The descriptions below focus on diagnostic clues to be found in the history (Figure 63) and neurological examination.

Hypoxia

Apathy may occur with hypotonia; hyperexcitability and fits with hypertonia. Occasionally there are unilateral neurological signs (hemisyndrome). A changing pattern is sometimes observed, e.g. apathy followed by hyperexcitability. The hypoxial insult may have occurred antepartum, intrapartum or more rarely postpartum. Events and circumstances suggestive of the occurrence of hypoxia should be specifically sought and the probability of hypoxia as a causal event carefully gauged. 'Hypoxia almost certain' would be applied to a neonate, monitored during labour, who had an abnormal fetal heart rate, fetal blood pH <7.1 and who required positive pressure ventilation at birth. A neonate with abnormal neurological behaviour who is merely 'at risk of hypoxia' (e.g.

the occurrence of antepartum bleeding) is just as likely to have other treatable conditions such as sepsis or a metabolic disturbance.

Birth Trauma

Mechanical birth trauma and intrapartum hypoxia often coexist as potent causes of abnormal neurological behaviour. The probability of birth trauma is easier to gauge by the nature of the delivery than that of hypoxia. Subdural haemorrhage is usually fatal and results from rupture of the great cerebral vein or tearing of a dural sinus. A clinical picture of a torn tentorium that is easily confused with congenital heart disease or a respiratory disorder is that of a cyanosed, bruised term baby with apathy, floppiness and irregular rapid respirations. Trauma to the cervical cord may occur during a difficult breech extraction. Apathy, floppiness and enlargement of the bladder associated with bladder paralysis has been described in affected neonates (De Souza and Davis 1974).

Maternally Administered Drugs

Apathy, impaired sucking and swallowing, respiratory depression and floppiness are prominent neurological features observed in newborn babies when mothers are overzealously 'treated' by certain sedative or analgesic drugs during labour. In contrast the accidental injection of local anaesthetic drugs into the fetus or their absorption from the maternal circulation is a cause of neonatal fits. Hyperexcitability and fits may occur as part of a withdrawal reaction in neonates of mothers addicted to drugs such as heroin, amphetamine and alcohol. Although symptoms usually occur within 24 hours, they can begin as late as two to three weeks, especially if methadone was taken by the mother.

Sepsis

Neonatal fits may be the only clinical feature of intra-uterine infections such as cytomegalovirus, rubella and toxoplasmosis. Rarely in such cases is there a clue to the presence of maternal infection in pregnancy, and the relevant investigations are prompted by failure to find an alternative cause for the fits. An apathetic, floppy neonate may have serious bacterial infection such as meningitis or septicaemia, and the prognosis is powerfully influenced by the promptness with which antibiotic therapy is started. Fortunately there may be important historical clues which alert the clinician to the presence of sepsis acquired by the ascending route *in utero* or postnatally (Figure 63).

Electrolyte and Metabolic Disturbances

Focal fits do not exclude metabolic or electrolyte disturbances as their aetiology. Jitteriness and focal, multifocal or generalised clonic fits may occur in association with hypocalcaemia and hypomagnesaemia. The most common type of symptomatic hypocalcaemia presents between the fifth and seventh day in babies fed on cows' milk. Hypomagnesaemia may co-exist (Chiswick 1971). In neonates, abnormally high or low plasma sodium levels occur with virtually any behaviour pattern including fits. Premature neonates receiving intravenous fluids are especially at risk. It is irrelevant to ponder on the clues which might prompt a diagnosis of symptomatic hypoglycaemia, because neonates with *any* type of abnormal neurological behaviour should have their blood glucose estimated by Dextrostix at once. Many different inborn errors of metabolism may present in the neonate with apathy and hypotonia or fits. Most are inherited as an autosomal recessive and the occurrence of an unexplained neonatal death in a sibling may provide a clue to this group of disorders. Other clues are shown in Figure 63.

Non-Traumatic Intracranial Haemorrhage

Intraventricular haemorrhage (IVH) and subarachnoid haemorrhage (SAH) are prone to occur in premature babies with idiopathic respiratory distress or recurrent apnoeic attacks. Thus apathy and floppiness is a common finding before the onset of the bleed, making clinical diagnosis notoriously difficult. In the author's experience the development of fits or hyperexcitability is uncommon and the prominent 'new' neurological feature is the sudden occurrence of diminished responsiveness to external stimulation in association with a sudden unexplained fall in the arterial Po_2, a falling blood pH and signs of peripheral circulatory failure. When impaired blood coagulation plays a significant role in the aetiology,

bleeding from the umbilical stump and puncture sites may be a clue to the diagnosis.

Structural Cerebral Defects

Unless there is a grossly abnormal result on transillumination of the skull, a structural cerebral defect should not be clinically considered in the absence of a major abnormality of the head or facies.

Congenital Neuromuscular Abnormalities

These abnormalities are relatively rare, and floppiness is a feature common to all of them. Twenty-five per cent of neonates born to mothers with myasthenia gravis have temporary myasthenia at or soon after birth, manifest by poor respiratory effort, weak cry, feeding difficulty and abnormal eye movements in addition to floppiness. The signs abate promptly when 1.0 mg edrophonium chloride (Tensilon) is given intravenously. Maintenance therapy is required for up to six weeks (1 to 5 mg neostigmine (Prostigmin) six hourly). Certain congenital myopathies are inherited as an autosomal dominant, whereas Werdnig–Hoffmann disease and glycogen storage disease of muscle are inherited as an autosomal recessive. There may be a history of poor fetal movements in Werdnig–Hoffmann disease and characteristically the tendon jerks are absent. However, apart from temporary myasthenia gravis, the precise diagnosis in this group of disorders

Figure 66. *Investigation of abnormal neurological behaviour.*

All babies	**Antepartum sepsis**	**Neuromuscular**
Blood glucose Plasma sodium Capillary pH Pco_2 Examine urine for smell and reducing substances (Clinistix *and* Clinitest) Bacterial infection screen including CSF, blood and urine culture Peripheral blood WBC (total and differential) Transilluminate skull	Serum IgM Viral culture (throat swab and urine) Serology Skull X-ray	Diagnostic IM injection of 1 mg Tensilon in floppy babies Muscle biopsy Electromyography Plasma creatine phosphokinase
	Electrolyte/metabolic Plasma calcium, magnesium, Amino acid chromatography Organic acid chromatography Plasma ammonia Diagnostic IV infusion of 25 mg pyridoxine if intractable fits occur	**Chromosomal** Lymphocyte culture and examination of chromosomes
		Role of EEG Not essential, but may be a useful adjunct in the assessment of prognosis
	Non-traumatic intracranial haemorrhage Note any blood-staining of CSF when the specimen is obtained for culture Blood coagulation studies	**Rarely indicated** Ventricular tap Subdural tap Air ventriculogram

rests on the results of muscle biopsy and electromyography. Neonates with persistent hypotonia of unexplained origin and those with a relevant family history should be referred to a centre with experience in the diagnosis of congenital neuromuscular disorders.

Investigation

It is unhelpful to perform numerous investigations in the hope that 'something will turn up'. It is important to begin by screening for treatable conditions. There is a minimum basic group of investigations which should be performed on all babies presenting with abnormal neurological behaviour (Figure 66). Although transillumination of the skull rarely reveals a treatable lesion, it should always be performed because the finding of a gross intracranial abnormality may obviate further investigations. The skull is systematically illuminated with a bright torch in a completely darkened room. Abnormalities such as subarachnoid cysts, subdural haematomata, hydrocephalus, hydranencephaly, porencephalic cysts and cerebral atrophy may be revealed as a halo of illumination extending more than 2.5 cm from the rim of the torch in the frontal region and more than 1 cm in the occipital region.

Other investigations shown in Figure 66 are prompted by knowledge of events and circumstances, and the nature of the abnormal signs and symptoms.

Treatment

Priority is given to the treatment of any underlying cause such as sepsis, or metabolic or electrolyte disturbance. Often a treatable cause is not found and therapy is directed towards the relief of symptoms (Table 39).

Prognosis

When a neonate exhibits abnormal neurological behaviour the prognosis for neurological or intellectual development is influenced by:

1. The cause of the disturbance.

2. The nature and evolution of signs and symptoms.

3. Genetic endowment.

4. Social environmental factors.

The prognosis is excellent, for example, when fits occur in association with hypocalcaemia towards the end of the first week, but much less optimistic when fits occur on the second day in association with hypoglycaemia. When a cause has not been found, the prognosis should be guarded in the following circumstances.

1. Convulsions occurring during the first two or three days of life.

2. The persistence of abnormal neurological features throughout the neonatal period.

Congenital Malformations of the CNS

The CNS is the most frequent site of congenital malformation. Anencephaly is the most frequent abnormality and those affected are usually stillborn. Three other abnormalities are briefly discussed below.

Microcephaly

An abnormally small head may be arbitrarily defined as one below the third centile when the OFC is plotted against age. The small head reflects an abnormally small brain and the majority of affected neonates become severely impaired developmentally. Microcephaly (Figure 67) may be present at birth or may gradually become apparent later, when for some reason (e.g. severe hypoxic brain damage at birth) the rate of head growth becomes abnormally slow. Examination of the brains of microcephalic infants shows that there is no uniform pattern of abnormality. Diverse findings such as gliosis, regional atrophy or agenesis, ventricular dilatation, etc., probably reflect the underlying causative insult.

Hydrocephalus

Hydrocephalus, an excess of cerebrospinal fluid within

Table 39. The relief of neurological symptoms.

1. Fits
Immediate treatment
paraldehyde 0.1 mg/kg IM
or
diazepam (Valium) 0.4 mg/kg IV (0.5 mg/min)
Maintenance therapy
phenobarbitone 5 to 7 mg/kg per day oral,
or IM 8 hourly
phenytoin (Epanutin) 4 to 8 mg/kg per day, oral or
IM 8 hourly.

2. Marked hyperexcitability
Chloral hydrate 60 mg/kg per day 8 hourly
or
phenobarbitone (see above)

3. Respiratory depression
Monitor respiration (e.g. use apnoea alarm mattress)
Appropriate ventilatory support if indicated

4. Raised intracranial pressure
Almost impossible to diagnose with certainty.
When a hypoxic insult is clearly the cause of gross apathy or hyperexcitability it is probably reasonable to use dexamethasone 1 mg IM 12 hourly for up to 3 days (gradually tail off dose).

Figure 67. *Congenital microcephaly.*

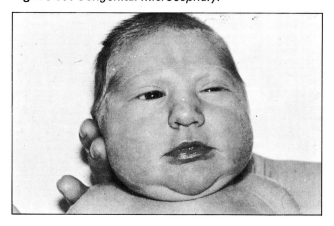

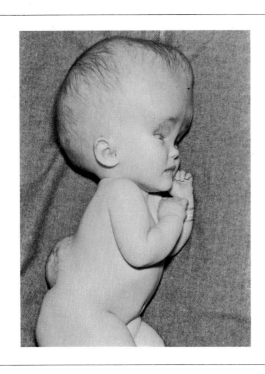

Figure 68. *Gross hydrocephalus rapidly developed after birth in this baby with a myelomeningocele.*

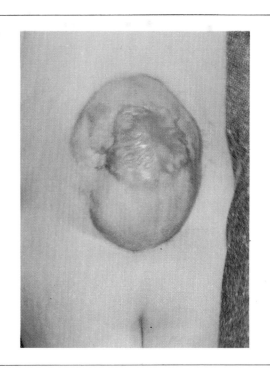

Figure 69. *In this example of a large myelomeningocele the neural plaque in the centre of the lesion is covered by a thin membrane.*

the ventricles and subarachnoid space, may be suspected at birth when the OFC is above the 97th centile. More commonly, it is suspected after birth by a rapid increase in head size such that the serial OFC plot crosses two centile lines. When this occurs in association with excess separation of the skull sutures, a tense anterior fontanelle or symptoms of raised intracranial pressure (vomiting, lethargy, fits), surgical intervention is necessary. Insertion of a shunt between the dilated ventricles and right atrium is one surgical approach.

The most common cause of hydrocephalus is the Arnold–Chiari malformation in association with a myelomeningocele (Figure 68). In this anomaly there is downward displacement and distortion of part of the medulla and cerebellum through the foramen magnum.

Myelomeningocele

The incidence of myelomeningocele in Western Europe is about three per thousand live births. A flat or raised neural plaque is exposed on the midline of the back and surrounded by a blueish membrane which merges with the skin (Figure 69). Very occasionally the lesion may be covered by skin (closed myelomeningocele). Although the lumbar region is the most common single site, involvement of adjacent areas is frequent, and in over 60 per cent of cases the lesion in thoracolumbar or thoracolumbar-sacral. The clinical problems commonly encountered are shown in Table 40. Neonatal assessment is helpful in indicating the minimal disability that can be expected, and the decision to close the lesion soon after birth and embark on a complicated programme of care is largely influenced by the findings. An excellent review of the neonatal assessment was given by Stark (1971). The

paediatric neurosurgeon will perform his own assessment, paying careful attention to the level and extent of the spinal lesion in terms of motor, sensory, bladder and bowel function. However, all those caring for the newborn should be able to make a preliminary assessment and provide 'on the spot' information to the neurosurgeon before he sees the baby (Table 41).

Before surgery the lesion should be covered with sterile gauze soaked in saline. Hydrocephalus usually develops rapidly after closure of the myelomeningocele. The head circumference should be measured twice weekly. Close liaison should be maintained with the neurosurgeon to ensure that a shunt operation is performed at the optimal time.

Traumatic Nerve Palsies

The most common lesions are of the facial nerve and brachial plexus.

Facial Nerve

The lesion is unilateral and may occur whether or not forceps were applied to the head. When the baby cries, the eye cannot be fully closed on the affected side and the nasolabial fold is absent. The mouth is drawn to the side of the lesion. Complete recovery usually occurs within a few weeks. Care of the exposed eye is important and methylcellulose drops should be instilled.

Brachial Plexus

The roots of the brachial plexus may be damaged during difficult deliveries, particularly breech extraction and shoulder impaction. A lesion of the upper roots (Erb's palsy) is the most common. The arm is adducted and in-

Table 40. Clinical problems encountered in myelomeningocele.

Various degrees of paralysis of lower limbs
Lower limb deformity
Kyphosis and/or scoliosis
Bladder paralysis
Impaired sphincter function
Hydrocephalus

Table 41. Preliminary assessment of a neonate with a myelomeningocele.

1. Note any history of intrapartum hypoxia or trauma.
2. Note birthweight and gestational age.
3. Measure the occipitofrontal head circumference.
4. Is the baby alert with a normal cry?
5. Note site and size of the lesion. Is there a complete covering membrane?
6. Is the lesion leaking CSF?
7. Is there kyphosis or scoliosis?
8. Note nature of limb movements.
9. Note nature of limb deformities.
10. Is there dribbling of urine? Is the bladder palpable?
11. Is the anus patulous? Does the external sphincter promptly contract in response to a light pin prick over the perianal skin?
12. Are there recognisable malformations outside the CNS?

Figure 70. *Neonate with Erb's palsy.*

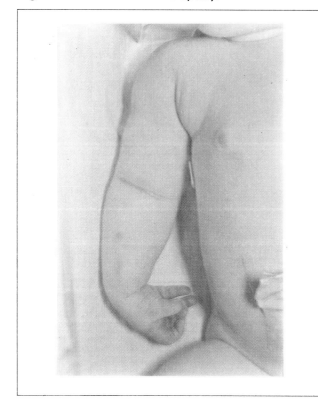

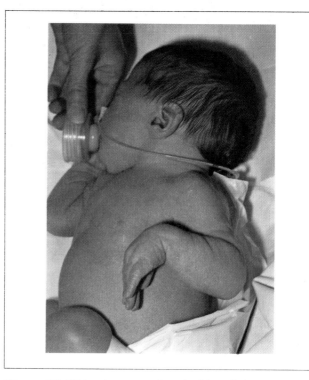

Figure 71. *Wrist drop associated with radial nerve palsy. A depression in the skin just visible overlying the anterolateral aspect of the humerus was probably caused by a constriction band in utero.*

palsy) is associated with wrist drop and flaccid paralysis of the hand. In some cases an area of fat necrosis or bruising is visible over the anterolateral aspect of the upper arm, overlying the radial groove of the humerus, and suggesting a lesion of the radial nerve rather than the lower roots of the brachial plexus (Figure 71).

The prognosis depends on the exact pathology of the lesion which, of course, is unknown. There must be a wide spectrum of injury ranging from minor contusion of nerve roots to complete avulsion from the spinal cord. Generally, when recovery occurs within six months it is total, but residual weakness is common when signs are present beyond six months. Treatment consists of gentle passive movements to the affected limb and supportive splints for the wrists and fingers when appropriate.

References

Baum, J. D. and Bulpitt, C. J., *Arch. Dis. Child.,* 1970, **45**, 344.
Chiswick, M. L., *Brit. Med. J.,* 1971, **3**, 15.
De Souza, S. W. and Davis, J. A., *Arch. Dis. Child.,* 1974, **49**, 70.
Prechtl, H. F. R. and Beintema, D., *The Neurological Examination of the Newborn Infant.* Clinics in Developmental Medicine, No. 12. SIMP and Heinemann, London, 1964.
Robinson, R. J., *Arch. Dis. Child.,* 1966, **41**, 437.
Stark, G., *Arch. Dis. Child.,* 1971, **46**, 539.

Further Reading

Saint-Anne Dargassies, S., *Neurological Development in the Full-Term and Premature Neonate,* Elsevier-North Holland, The Netherlands, 1977.

ternally rotated at the shoulder. The elbow is extended with the forearm pronated. Wrist flexion with finger extension also occurs giving the 'waiter's tip' posture (Figure 70). Occasionally there is an associated diaphragmatic paralysis. A lesion of the lower roots (Klumpke's

10. Gastrointestinal Problems

GASTROINTESTINAL signs and symptoms that may be observed in the neonate include vomiting, abdominal distension, diarrhoea, failure to pass meconium within 24 hours of birth, and the passage of blood-stained stools (see Figure 72).

Vomiting is the most common of these disturbances and is selected for discussion. The diagnostic approach to vomiting suggested below serves as a framework which may be modified for other gastrointestinal signs and symptoms which occasionally dominate the clinical picture.

Vomiting

Although sometimes observed in a benign form in normal babies, vomiting is a feature of such diverse conditions as congenital alimentary tract obstruction, sepsis or inborn errors of metabolism. At the first consultation certain features in the history that might provide a clue to the diagnosis must be carefully noted. During subsequent consultations the clinician is then free to focus carefully on the progress of the symptoms and the development of new signs and symptoms.

Family history. Certain types of alimentary tract obstruction and metabolic disorders are genetically determined.

Hydramnios. A history of maternal hydramnios is present in about 50 per cent of neonates with oesophageal, duodenal or jejunal atresia.

Birth history. Birth asphyxia and cerebral trauma are potent causes of cerebral oedema and intracranial haemorrhage. Vomiting may dominate the abnormal neurological signs and occur soon after birth or be delayed from 24 to 48 hours. Do not hastily attribute vomiting to asphyxial or traumatic events during birth, because alimentary tract malformation, sepsis or inborn errors of metabolism may each occur in neonates who have suffered from a degree of asphyxia or cerebral trauma.

Nature of the vomiting. The presence of bile in the vomitus means intestinal obstruction until otherwise proven, whereas the absence of bile does not rule out obstruction which may be present above the ampulla of Vater. Projectile vomiting does not invariably occur in obstruction and babies who vomit milk as they burp may do so with considerable force. In lower bowel obstruction the onset of vomiting may be delayed beyond 24 hours. Do

Vomiting	Abdominal Distension
Benign vomiting	Alimentary tract
Alimentary tract	obstruction
obstruction	Functional ileus
Functional ileus	Necrotising enterocolitis
Necrotising enterocolitis	Peritonitis
Peritonitis	Stomach distension
Hiatus hernia	during assisted ventilation
Sepsis, including	Massive pneumothorax
gastroenteritis	Enlarged abdominal organ
Cerebral oedema	Tumours and cysts
Intracranial haemorrhage	Ascites
Inborn errors of metabolism	Disaccharide intolerance
Renal insufficiency	
Diarrhoea	**Blood in Stools**
Sepsis including	Swallowed maternal
gastroenteritis	blood
Necrotising enterocolitis	Haemorrhagic disease of
Disaccharide intolerance	the newborn
Cystic fibrosis	Injury by rectal
Maternal laxatives in	thermometer
breast milk	Anal fissure
Maternal drug addiction	Necrotising enterocolitis
Congenital adrenal	Bacterial peritonitis
hyperplasia	Volvulus
Congenital thyrotoxicosis	Duplication of the
	intestine

Figure 72. *Some causes of common gastrointestinal signs and symptoms in the neonate.*

not be complacent about intermittent vomiting. It may indicate incomplete obstruction.

Passage of stools. Vomiting should never be attributed to a benign cause when there is an associated disturbance of bowel function. Watery or abnormally loose stools occur in a wide spectrum of disorders including infective gastroenteritis, necrotising enterocolitis, septicaemia and inborn errors of metabolism. Vomiting in association with a delay beyond 24 hours in the passage of meconium is a feature of bowel obstruction. However, many neonates with a high or partial obstruction do pass meconium on the first day of life. The stools should be inspected with special attention to the presence of blood (Figure 72).

Behaviour pattern. Never assume a benign cause for vomiting when reluctance to feed, lethargy or hyperexcitability is present.

Examination

A general examination should always be performed before focusing on the abdomen. Conversely, when a baby presents late and vomiting in association with a primary gastrointestinal disorder has contributed to circulatory collapse, the unwary may easily neglect the abdomen as the source of the problem. In this respect peritonitis in a severely ill neonate can be readily overlooked. The state of hydration must be carefully assessed (Table 41). The baby should be weighed to compare with previous weights and a baseline established for future measurements. The following features should be specifically sought on abdominal examination.

Abdominal distension. Some causes of abdominal distension are shown in Figure 72. Vomiting never has a benign cause when abdominal distension is present. When in doubt about the presence of this sign, protrusion of the navel or undue fullness at the base of the umbilical cord stump suggests that the abdomen is distended. Ascertain whether the distension is localised or generalised. Measure the abdominal girth at the level of the umbilicus so that the physical sign can be serially and objectively assessed.

Skin overlying abdomen. In a series of 91 cases of neonatal peritonitis, skin discoloration and oedema of the abdominal wall was a feature of one-third (Rickham and Johnston 1969). When the abdomen is greatly distended the overlying skin frequently appears stretched and shiny, and venous tributaries are prominent.

Visible peristalsis is frequently seen in otherwise normal pre-term or small-for-dates neonates who have a thin abdominal wall. In conjunction with vomiting and abdominal distension this suggests alimentary tract obstruction.

Palpation and percussion. Pay careful attention to enlargement of viscera (liver, spleen, kidneys, bladder) as well as the presence of abnormal masses (abscess, duplication cysts, Wilms' tumour, neuroblastoma, etc.). Assess the degree of resonance of the distended abdomen by percussion. Fluid in the peritoneal cavity may be revealed by the conventional test for shifting dullness and a fluid thrill. Guarding on palpation is not invariably present in peritonitis, particularly when the baby is very ill.

Rectal examination. Confirm the presence of an anal opening and note whether it is normally positioned. In neonates with vomiting and abdominal distension, rectal examination may suggest Hirschsprung's disease when a

gush of meconium and flatus and relief of distension occurs soon after the examining finger is withdrawn. A narrow empty rectum is commonly found in Hirschsprung's disease, necrotising enterocolitis and peritonitis.

Inspect the hernial orifices.

Observe the baby feeding. Finally, the cause of the vomiting may be apparent by observation of the feeding technique. If the baby's clinical state justifies the procedure an oral feed should be observed in the natural setting.

Investigation

The appropriate investigations obviously vary in individual neonates, but the following tests should never be omitted in ill neonates with unexplained vomiting.

Blood Electrolytes, Urea and pH

Although neonates may rapidly develop severe disturbances of electrolyte balance as a result of vomiting, it should be remembered that hyponatraemia often occurs insidiously, particularly in low birthweight babies who may vomit only small amounts of milk over a long period.

Occasionally results give a clue to the aetiology. A metabolic acidosis that is severe in relation to the extent of the vomiting might suggest an inborn error of metabolism. Significant hyponatraemia in association with hyperkalaemia occurs in the salt-losing variety of congenital adrenal hyperplasia. The blood urea concentration in the neonate is powerfully influenced by the protein intake and is a poor guide to the state of hydration. However, a marked increase in the blood urea out of proportion to the signs of dehydration suggests a primary renal problem (e.g. hypoplastic kidneys, pyelonephritis, obstructive uropathy).

Blood Glucose

Hypoglycaemia is liable to occur in any ill neonate but particularly when vomiting is associated with a reduced milk intake. Vomiting and hypoglycaemia are features of galactosaemia and other inborn errors of metabolism—a group of disorders readily overlooked.

Ward Testing of Urine

Simple tests may give a clue to the presence of inborn errors of metabolism. Note whether the urine has an abnormal smell. A positive 'Clinitest' yet a negative 'Clinistix' may occur in galactosaemia. Ketonuria (detected by 'Acetest') with keto-aciduria (a precipitate occurs in four to five minutes when one volume of a saturated solution of 2, 4 dinitrophenolhydrazine in hydrochloric acid is added drop wise to a half volume of urine) is a feature of the organic acidaemias.

Bacterial Infection Screen

It is impossible to rule out by clinical examination bacterial sepsis as a cause of neonatal vomiting. When functional ileus occurs in association with sepsis, the clinical picture may be confused with congenital bowel obstruction. Also septicaemia sometimes occurs in peritonitis

Table 41. Signs of dehydration.

Abnormal weight loss.
Poor urinary output.
Loss of skin turgor.
Dry skin.
Depressed anterior fontanelle.
Sunken eyes.

and necrotising enterocolitis. Investigations should include a total and differential white cell count, culture of superficial swabs, blood, urine and cerebrospinal fluid.

Abdominal X-ray

An erect and supine plain X-ray of the abdomen may suggest the presence of alimentary tract obstruction, bowel perforation, ascites, necrotising enterocolitis, or may delineate a mass. Swallowed air reaches the intestine within an hour of birth and the anus by 3 to 12 hours. Observation of the distribution of air and fluid levels within the alimentary tract may suggest not only the presence of obstruction but also the site and degree, i.e. whether partial or complete. The use of swallowed radio-opaque dyes for this purpose is rarely necessary. The role of the plain abdominal X-ray in the diagnosis of gastrointestinal pathology is illustrated in Figures 73, 76 to 79 and 81.

Management

Regardless of the cause, when vomiting is persistent or associated with an electrolyte disturbance or signs of dehydration, oral feeding should be stopped and fluids given intravenously via a peripheral vein. Priority is given to the treatment of peripheral circulatory failure, when present, by an infusion of plasma or 0.9 per cent saline (30 ml/kg during one half to one hour). The total volume required for the correction of fluid deficit may be roughly assessed by knowledge of abnormal weight loss (100 ml needed for each 100 g weight loss) or by the degree of clinical dehydration (Table 42). An additional allowance is required for maintenance (100 to 150 ml/kg/day) and on-going abnormal losses when present (e.g. aspirated stomach contents, diarrhoea). The plasma sodium concentration is an important guide to the concentration of saline solution to be infused.

Any regime of electrolyte replacement must be modified in the light of frequent clinical assessments and the results of blood electrolyte analysis.

Special Problems

Certain medical and surgical problems of the gastrointestinal tract with special implications are briefly discussed below.

Medical Problems

Benign Vomiting

The poor terminology is only justified if it reminds the clinician that what is benign clinically may be a source of much worry to a mother who often sees her care-giver role as that of a milk provider first. Naturally she is distressed when her bounty is rejected. The term is applicable to healthy neonates who vomit from time to time and who do not have abnormal weight loss or clinical signs. There are probably many different causes. Babies often eject a small amount of milk as they are burped. Small vomits in the first day or two of life that are self-limiting are often attributed to 'mucous gastritis' implying that excess amounts of swallowed mucus may irritate the stomach. The traditional gastric lavage that is performed for this condition in many maternity hospitals is probably unjustified. Incoordinate oesophageal action and delayed gastric emptying may also contribute to benign vomiting.

Sometimes a mother makes many unnecessary changes of position of the baby during a feed—an experience that many an adult stomach would object to violently. A mother should be given the opportunity to discuss her problem thoroughly with a doctor or nurse who has a sympathetic understanding of the situation. When the relationship between the mother and her newborn baby is upset, even transiently, it will not be easily forgotten by either party.

Infective Gastroenteritis

Note that in some cases the stools are so watery that they may be absorbed by the napkin and mistaken for urine. Many specimens of stools may have to be cultured before the responsible organism (e.g. pathogenic *E. coli*, shigella, salmonella species) is identified. Symptoms of gastroenteritis often abate without an offending organism being identified. Mild diarrhoea often ceases when the milk feeds are temporarily diluted with sterile water for 24 to 48 hours.

If significant vomiting occurs or signs of dehydration are present, oral feeding should be temporarily discontinued and intravenous fluids substituted. Occasionally a recurrence of diarrhoea occurs when milk feeds are reintroduced because of transient lactose intolerance. In such instances a lactose-free milk should be used. Parenteral antibiotics should be given because it is not possible to exclude clinically an associated septicaemia. Precautions must be taken to prevent the spread of transmissible bowel pathogens through the neonatal nursery (Table 43).

Necrotising Enterocolitis

Necrotising enterocolitis has a predilection for low birth weight babies, especially those who have suffered hypoxic episodes and those subjected to umbilical arterial or venous catheterisation, particularly for exchange transfusion. Symptoms and signs include vomiting, the passage of loose stools which are often blood-stained, unstable body temperature, apnoeic attacks and abdominal distension. The abdominal X-ray appearance early on is of moderately dilated bowel loops that may have thickened (oedematous) walls. Subsequently, linear streaks of intra-

Table 42. Volume of IV fluid required for the correction of dehydration.

Clinical degree of dehydration	Mild	Moderate	Severe
Per cent weight loss	5	10	15
Volume required (ml/per kg normal body weight)	50	100	150

N.B. Rehydration should be completed in 24 hours.

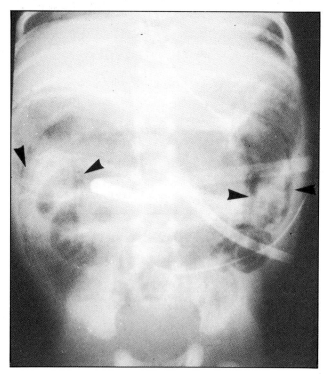
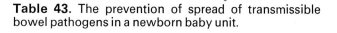

Figure 73a. *Necrotising enterocolitis. Linear translucencies outline the wall of the dilated bowel seen on the right and left side of the abdomen.*

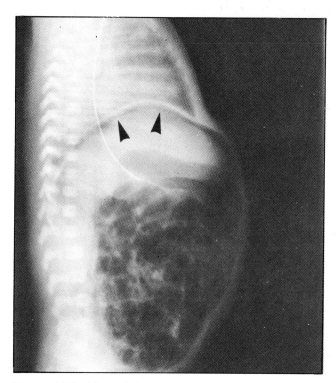

Figure 73b. *Necrotising enterocolitis complicated by bowel perforation. In the lateral erect view of the abdomen free gas is visible under the diaphragm, and the bowel is distended.*

Table 43. The prevention of spread of transmissible bowel pathogens in a newborn baby unit.

Remove mother and baby to a ward where there are no newborn babies and where there is adequate nursing and medical staff supervision.

Restrict nursing care to nurses who do not deal with other infants or work in a milk kitchen.

Take special care in the disposal of napkins or other items removed from the baby.

Consult with the bacteriologist about arrangements for tracing the source of infection.

Until the source is traced and eradicated it may be necessary to close the unit to new admissions.

The family doctor should be informed of the occurrence of nursery infections when apparently well babies are discharged to his care.

mural air become visible (Figure 73a), and the portal venous system within the liver may be partially outlined by air. The presence of gas under the diaphragm indicates that bowel perforation has occurred (Figure 73b). The aetiology is unknown, but gut ischaemia in association with a disturbed bacterial flora in the bowel plays a role.

However, a prevalence of gas-forming organisms on stool culture is only occasionally observed. It is noteworthy that the condition is rare in wholly breast-fed neonates. Treatment includes the substitution of intravenous fluids for milk, gastric aspiration and parenteral antibiotics (e.g. penicillin and gentamycin). Bowel per-

foration is an indication for surgery. Extensive gangrene of the bowel requiring resection is frequently found.

Surgical Problems

Details of surgical treatment are only briefly mentioned. However it is important to be aware of certain principles when referring a neonate to the surgical unit of another hospital. When the mother cannot accompany the baby, ensure that she knows exactly where her baby is going, i.e. name of hospital, ward and telephone number. A specimen of maternal blood should accompany the baby, because this may be used in cross-matching should the baby require a transfusion.

Ensure that the mother has an opportunity to see and touch her baby before transfer. Do not just whisk away her offspring. Make sure that the surgeon is aware of the baby's general condition before transfer because he may be able to offer facilities to collect and safely transport the baby to his unit using specially trained staff. The stomach contents must be intermittently or continuously aspirated when there is alimentary tract obstruction. Correction of circulatory failure, hypoglycaemia and acidosis and the prevention of abnormal heat loss are essential considerations before the neonate is transferred.

Exomphalos

Exomphalos is a congenital herniation of some of the intra-abdominal contents through the umbilical ring (Figure 74). The herniation is covered by a membrane of amnion and peritoneum separated by Wharton's jelly.

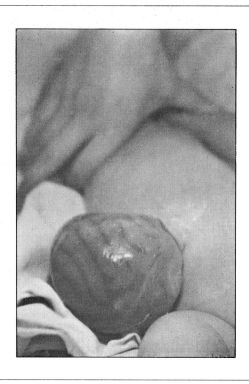

Figure 74. *Exomphalos. Loops of bowel are seen through the glistening hernial sac. The umbilical vessels are contained within the wall of the sac.*

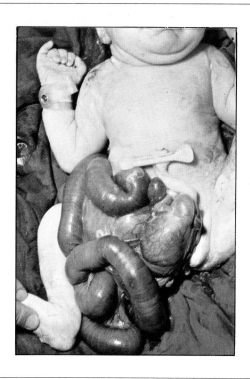

Figure 75. *Gastroschisis. Gangrenous bowel and stomach are seen protruded through a defect in the abdominal wall adjacent to the umbilicus.*

The size of the lesion is variable and coils of intestine may be visible through the membrane before it becomes relatively opaque several hours after birth. There are associated malformations of the gastrointestinal, genitourinary and cardiovascular system in about 40 per cent of cases, and an association of macroglossia with exomphalos has been well documented.

Immediate treatment consists of covering the lesion with wet sterile dressings and aspirating the stomach every ten minutes to prevent vomiting and abdominal distention. If the lesion is small, the sac can be excised, the viscera returned to the abdominal cavity and the defect in the anterior abdominal wall closed in one stage. However, in large lesions the abdominal cavity is too small to hold all the intestine. The skin may have to be closed over the exomphalos until the abdominal cavity has grown sufficiently to allow the hernia to be reduced. The average mortality is 50 per cent.

Gastroschisis

Coils of intestine and sometimes the stomach are eviscerated through a defect in the abdominal wall adjacent to the umbilicus (Figure 75). Associated malformations are uncommon. The intestinal circulation is always impaired and occasionally frank gangrene is observed. Preoperative management is similar to that outlined for exomphalos. Return of the herniated bowel to the small abdominal cavity is rarely possible. An alternative is to close the widely undermined skin of the abdominal wall over the lesion. The mortality is very high.

Congenital Alimentary Tract Obstruction

In cases of congenital alimentary tract obstruction any site may be involved. The obstruction may be partial or complete. Different types of obstructions occur including atresia, stenosis, intraluminal obstruction of the intestine by meconium, compression from outside (e.g. the presence of bands in association with malrotation of the intestine), and functional abnormalities of the bowel wall (e.g. Hirschsprung's disease). Vomiting, abdominal distension and delayed passage of meconium should alert the doctor or nurse to the possibility of some sort of congenital obstruction.

Congenital pyloric stenosis is not truly congenital but may first present towards the end of the neonatal period. Boys, particularly the first born, are more commonly affected than girls, and there is a familial predilection. Characteristically, projectile vomiting occurs after feeds and is associated with constipation. Immediately after vomiting the baby will often take another feed eagerly. When diagnosis is delayed, weight loss, dehydration and a hypochloraemic alkalosis are common features. Abdominal examination during a feed reveals visible peristalsis across the epigastrium from left to right, and an olive-shaped firm tumour can be identified at the outer border of the right rectus muscle above the umbilicus. Projectile vomiting is observed during or soon after completion of the feed. At operation the hypertrophied and gritty pyloric muscle is split without incising the mucous membrane.

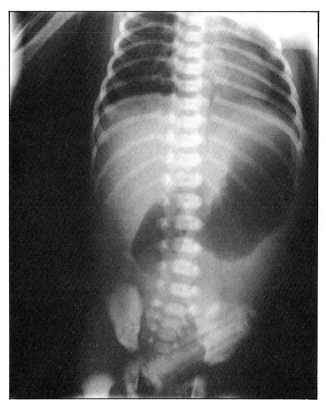

Figure 76. *Duodenal atresia showing the characteristic 'double bubble' appearance in the erect abdominal X-ray. The bubbles of air are in the stomach and dilated proximal part of the duodenum. No air has passed beyond a complete duodenal obstruction in this 24 hour old neonate.*

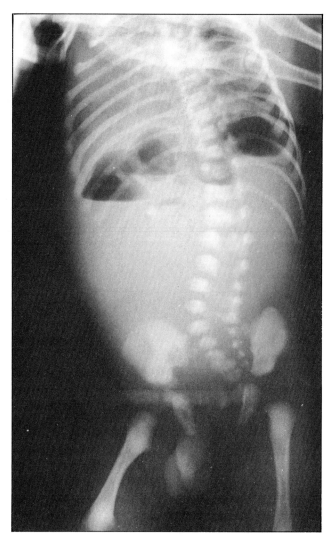

Figure 77. *Jejunal atresia. The erect abdominal X-ray shows many fluid levels in the dilated duodenum and jejunum proximal to an atretic segment beyond which air has failed to pass. This baby also had multiple abnormalities outside the gastrointestinal tract.*

Intestinal atresia and stenosis. Partial or complete obstruction may occur at any site from the duodenum to the colon. Duodenal obstruction usually occurs in the region of the ampulla of Vater. Associated major anomalies are common, including Down's syndrome, malrotation of the mid-gut and congenital heart disease. Obstruction of the intestine distal to the duodenum is less frequently associated with other anomalies but probably carries a greater risk of perforation and peritonitis. The higher the obstruction the earlier the onset of vomiting and the less marked is abdominal distension. Bile-stained vomitus is to be expected when the obstruction is below the ampulla of Vater.

While delay in the passage of meconium is particularly common, the passage of small amounts in the first 24 hours may occur even when obstruction is complete. Incomplete obstruction may not be suspected until several weeks after birth because of variability of signs and symptoms. A plain abdominal X-ray usually confirms that obstruction is present and points to the site (Figures 76 and 77).

Malrotation of the intestine. In the commonest type, adhesions (Ladd's bands) run across the duodenum from an abnormally high caecum to the parietal peritoneum in the right hypochondrium. Associated malformations include duodenal atresia or stenosis and exomphalos. The presenting features are those of duodenal obstruction but, because the obstruction is incomplete, mild signs and symptoms may be overlooked initially.

Meconium ileus. Meconium ileus occurs in certain neonates who have cystic fibrosis, a condition inherited as an autosomal recessive. Deficiency of pancreatic enzymes is associated with the occurrence of tenacious or inspissated meconium which obstructs the intestine. Gangrene of the bowel, perforation and meconium peritonitis are not uncommon complications. The clinical features are those of low intestinal obstruction with bile-stained vomiting, often marked abdominal distension and delay or failure to pass meconium. Stools of putty-like consistency are sometimes felt on abdominal examination. Abdominal X-ray shows markedly dilated bowel loops, although fluid levels may not be prominent (Figure 78).

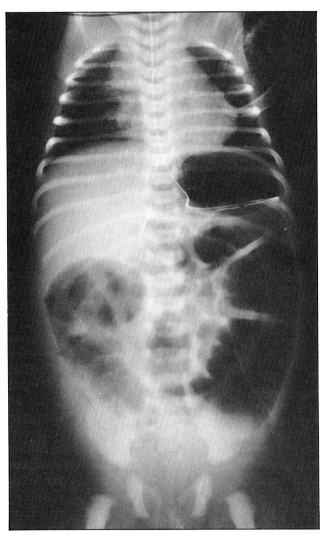

Figure 78. *Meconium ileus. Grossly dilated loops of small intestine with a virtual absence of fluid levels are seen in this erect abdominal X-ray. No gas is visible in the pelvis. At operation the small intestine was obstructed by tenacious meconium.*

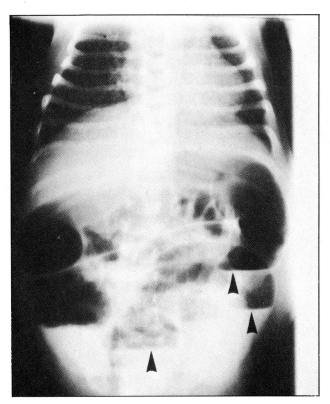

Figure 79. *Hirschsprung's disease. Grossly dilated loops of large bowel with many fluid levels are seen in this erect abdominal X-ray.*

Figure 80. *Anorectal atresia with rectovaginal fistula. The probe points to meconium passed* per vagina.

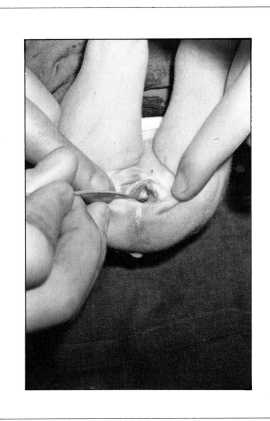

Hirschsprung's disease. An aganglionic segment of bowel extends for a variable distance in a proximal direction from the anal canal. Short segment disease is more common in males than females, whereas when a considerable length of the bowel is affected there is an equal sex distribution. There is a familial predilection. Symptoms are usually those of low intestinal obstruction and may present in the first 24 hours or be delayed for several days. Attention has previously been drawn to the findings on rectal examination. Plain abdominal X-ray confirms the presence of intestinal obstruction (Figure 79). A radio-opaque enema is required to show the narrowed aganglionic segment distal to the dilated bowel. The diagnosis is confirmed by histological examination of rectal biopsy material. Enterocolitis is a well-recognised complication of Hirschsprung's disease.

Anorectal malformations. Numerous different anomalies may occur. Rectal atresia as an isolated anomaly is uncommon. Usually the anus, anal canal and lower rectum

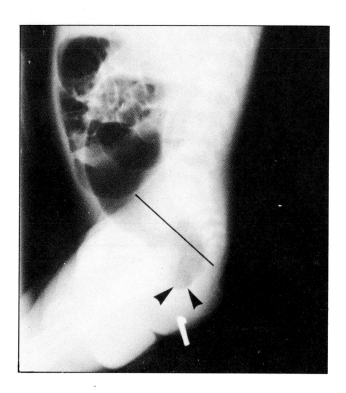

Figure 81. *'Covered anus'. The baby did not have an anal opening. A marker indicates the normal position of the anus in this lateral abdominal X-ray taken with the baby inverted. Note the terminal air shadow (arrowed) is distal to the pubococcygeal line indicating a 'low' anomaly, with a normal rectum.*

are absent and a fistula runs from the upper rectal pouch to the bladder, urethra or vagina (Figure 80). An obvious abnormality is therefore apparent on inspection of the perineum and signs of large bowel obstruction occur only if the fistula is small or not patent. Anal anomalies do not always involve the rectum. For example, an ectopic anus may be sited in the vaginal vestibule or anterior to its usual position (perineal anus).

In 'covered anus' the anal opening is absent and a fistula runs from the anal canal to the fourchette of the vagina or to a midline point between the frenulum of the prepuce and the perineum in the male. Occasionally the fistula opens into the urethra in the male. Finally the anal canal may simply be occluded by a membrane at the level of the anal valves. The important therapeutic and prognostic implication is to distinguish 'high' anomalies which involve the rectum from 'low' lesions. A lateral abdominal X-ray is taken for this purpose with the baby inverted. The site of the terminal gas bubble in relation to a line drawn from the pubis to the sacrococcygeal junction distinguishes 'high' from 'low' anomalies (Figure 81).

Reference

Rickham, P. P. and Johnston, J. H., *Neonatal Surgery,* page 355, Butterworth & Co. Ltd., London, 1969.

Further Reading

Koop, C. E., Schnaufer, L. and Broennie, A. M., *Pediatrics,* 1974, **54,** 558.

11. Genito-urinary Problems

THE function of the fetal kidneys is to provide an adequate quantity of urine for the maintenance of amniotic fluid volume. Biochemical homeostasis of the fetus is dependent on placental function, as illustrated by the finding of normal plasma urea and electrolyte levels at birth in babies with bilateral renal agenesis. The kidney of a newborn baby at term has its full complement of about 1,000,000 nephrons, but their functional capacity is much lower with respect to glomerular filtration, and particularly tubular reabsorption, than that of adult nephrons. Whilst renal function is adjusted to the anabolic or growth needs of the neonate, at the same time it limits the neonate's capacity to respond to the metabolic effects of many severe diseases, e.g. sepsis and the respiratory distress syndrome.

The manner of presentation of renal and urinary tract disease in the neonate is shown in Table 44.

Table 44. Presentation of renal problems in the neonate.

Nonspecific signs and symptoms of renal infection or renal insufficiency:
    jaundice
    lethargy
    poor feeding
    vomiting
    diarrhoea
    unstable body temperature
    abnormal weight loss
    dehydration

Palpable abdominal mass:
    hydronephrosis
    infantile polycystic disease
    multicystic kidney
    megacystis
    Wilms' tumour

Disorders of micturition:
    dribbling micturition
    failure to pass urine in first 24 hours (often an erroneous observation)

Visible abnormality:
    exstrophy of bladder
    epispadias
    hypospadias

Malpositions and Duplications

Horseshoe kidneys are fused at the lower pole and connected by an isthmus of renal parenchyma or fibrous tissue. One or both kidneys may be ectopic. A kidney may be ectopic on its own side (e.g. situated in the pelvis) or may cross the midline. Malpositioned kidneys are often asymptomatic but in certain situations, e.g. crossed renal ectopia, there is a real risk of ureteric obstruction and pyelonephritis.

Whereas the presence of more than two separate kidneys is a pathological rarity, duplication of the ureters and renal pelvis is a common anomaly. This would be a relatively harmless variation were it not sometimes accompanied by other anomalies. In the female, for example, the ureter draining the upper renal pelvis may terminate in the vagina or distal urethra causing urinary incontinence. In both sexes a duplicated ureter may drain into the trigone or bladder neck, terminating as an intravesical cyst or ectopic ureterocele. The affected ureter readily becomes obstructed, leading to hydronephrosis and predisposing to renal infection. Sometimes the obstructed segment of kidney is dysplastic (see below), suggesting that the obstructive lesion was present relatively early in gestation.

Hypospadias

The urethral meatus is situated on the ventral aspect of the penis proximal to its normal position. The orifice may be glandular, coronal, penile or penoscrotal, indicating that a varying length of urethra is absent. The following points are fundamental:

1. Meatal stenosis is present in about 25 per cent of cases.

2. The prepuce fails to unite ventrally (hooded prepuce).

3. Chordee, or ventral curvature of the penis, is present to different degrees.

4. A neonate with hypospadias should not be circumcized, because the prepuce may be utilized subsequently for operative repair of the lesion.

5. Hypospadias in association with undescended testes may be a manifestation of intersex.

Generally glandular or coronal hypospadias causes little problem apart from the occasional occurrence of meatal stenosis which is corrected by dilatation or meatotomy. In other forms, if left untreated, standing micturition is impossible and chordee renders sexual intercourse difficult. Operative treatment is generally performed in more than one stage with correction of the chordee preceding reconstruction of the terminal urethra. Ideally the repair should be completed just prior to school age.

Epispadias

This is quite different from hypospadias in that the urethra is present to the tip of the penis but is unroofed and exposed as a trough in the dorsal aspect of the penis. It is much less common than hypospadias and usually involves the whole length of the penis. There is usually an associated sphincteric defect and dribbling incontinence (Williams 1971). Rarely females are affected and in these cases the two halves of a split clitoris are situated on either side of a urethral strip. In the male, successful repair requires adequate penile size and generally this is feasible by the age of two to three years.

Exstrophy of the Bladder

This is a rare and serious anomaly that is invariably associated with epispadias and is more common in males. The pubic bones are widely separated and the vesical mucosa of the bladder is exposed through a defect in the lower anterior abdominal wall. There are numerous different approaches to operative treatment that have been modified with the passage of time, including total reconstruction in the neonatal period (Johnston 1970) or later and cystectomy and urinary diversion. Probably less than 30 per cent of males ultimately achieve urinary continence and freedom from urinary tract infection following reconstructive surgery. The outlook is somewhat better in females.

Structural Abnormalities of the Urinary Tract

Bilateral Renal Agenesis

The majority of affected babies are males and the lesion is relatively common, occurring in one out of 4,000 births. Most cases are sporadic, and stillbirth, intrauterine growth retardation and prematurity are common accompaniments. A history of maternal oligohydramnios is usual. There is a characteristic facial appearance (Potter's facies) with low-set malformed ears, a prominent skin fold below the eyes, a small chin and a beaked nose. The frequent occurrence of bow legs and club feet is attributed to the small liquor volume causing a postural defect *in utero* (Figure 82). Approximately 40 per cent of affected babies are stillborn and most of the others die soon after birth with respiratory distress secondary to pulmonary hypoplasia.

Renal Dysplasia

This term includes a broad spectrum of parenchymatous malformation ranging from a hypoplastic kidney so small as to be barely recognizable to a grossly enlarged kidney with cyst formation, i.e. multicystic kidney (Figure 83). One or both kidneys may be affected. The majority of dysplastic kidneys are associated with other anomalies of the renal tract and the multicystic kidney is commonly associated with ureteral atresia and pyelocalyceal occlusion. The pathogenesis of renal dysplasia is poorly understood but is probably related to an insult at the time of early renal differentiation in fetal life. Malformations in other systems, particularly the cardiovascular system and alimentary tract, are common. One important implication of renal dysplasia is vulnerability to pyelonephritis leading to scarring, atrophy and progressive renal impairment. Bilateral multicystic kidneys should not be confused with infantile polycystic disease.

Infantile Polycystic Disease

Both kidneys are always involved and they are diffusely enlarged with preservation of renal shape in contrast to multicystic kidneys (Figure 84a and b). The collecting tubules are dilated and are the site of numerous cysts. Macroscopically a cut section of kidney has a characteristic sponge-like appearance (Figure 84c). Polycystic changes are also present in the liver. The disease appears as a sporadic malformation or is inherited as an autosomal recessive. It has no relation to the adult type of polycystic disease which is inherited as an autosomal dominant. Infantile polycystic disease is usually suspected when bilateral renal masses are palpated. The majority of those affected are stillborn or die within the first few days of life. Those surviving the neonatal period suffer from gradually increasing renal impairment often complicated by systemic hypertension. Older children develop hepatic fibrosis, portal hypertension, hypersplenism and oesophageal varices.

Urinary Tract Obstruction

Hydronephrosis, or dilatation of the renal pelvis, is generally indicative of urinary tract obstruction and the lesion may be unilateral or bilateral. Obstruction in the upper urinary tract most frequently occurs at the ureteropelvic junction (e.g. stricture or aberrant vessel) or at the ureterovesical junction (e.g. stricture). Bilateral hydronephrosis may be associated with lower urinary tract obstruction (e.g. posterior urethral valves). Hydronephrosis also occurs without an obvious anatomical obstruction when the cause remains speculative. Regardless of the aetiology, urinary infection is common and a hydronephrotic mass may be converted into a bag of pus (pyelonephrosis).

The presenting feature may be the presence of an abdominal mass or nonspecific signs and symptoms of renal infection, or in bilateral cases, renal failure. Occasionally hydronephrotic kidneys and dilated tortuous ureters are associated with a congenital absence of the musculature of the anterior abdominal wall or 'prunebelly syndrome' (Figure 85). Intravenous pyelography often fails to visualize the hydronephrotic kidney. However, retrograde pyelography clearly demonstrates

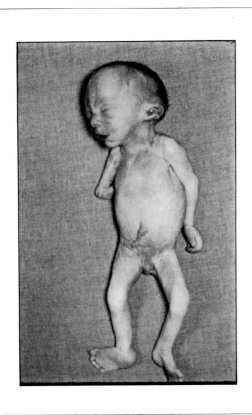

Figure 82. *Potter's syndrome, showing characteristic facial appearance and postural deformity of right foot.*

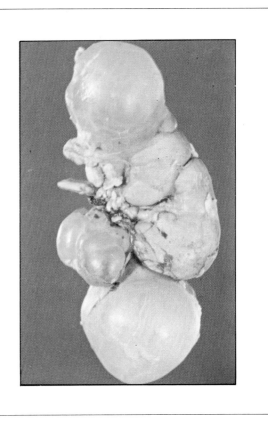

Figure 83. *Grossly enlarged kidney with multiple cyst formation, i.e. multicystic kidney.*

Figure 84a. *Infantile polycystic disease showing bilateral renal enlargement with overall preservation of renal shape and hepatomegaly.*

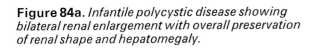

Figure 84b. *Infantile polycystic disease showing numerous cysts visible on surface of kidney.*

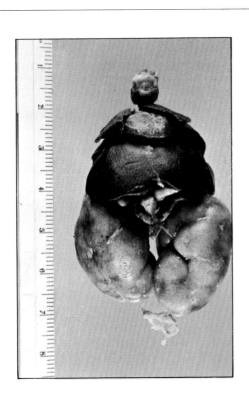

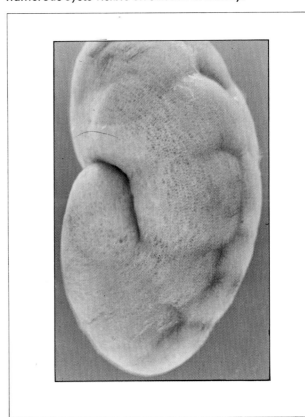

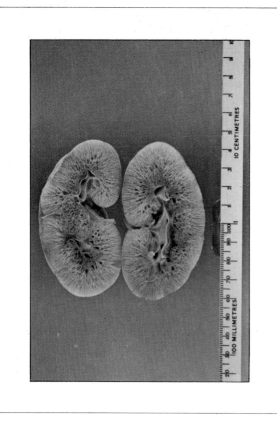

Figure 84c. *Infantile polycystic disease; cut section of kidney showing cystic appearance.*

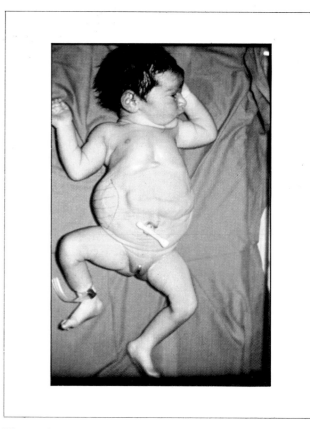

Figure 85. *Congenital absence of musculature of anterior abdominal wall in association with a hydronephrotic kidney on the right side.*

the dilated pelvis, clubbing of the calyces and perhaps ureteric dilatation and tortuosity (Figure 86). Treatment and prognosis depend on many factors, including the nature of any obstruction and its potential reversibility, whether the lesion is unilateral or bilateral, and the presence of urinary tract infection. Posterior urethral valves will be considered in more detail as an illustration of lower urinary tract obstruction.

Posterior Urethral Valves

This condition is virtually confined to male neonates. Mucosal valves pass downwards and laterally from the verumontanum and unite anteriorly causing obstruction to urinary flow. The bladder becomes hypertrophied and trabeculated and cysto-ureteric reflux occurs. The ureters are commonly dilated and tortuous and bilateral hydronephrosis is a frequent occurrence with urinary infection and functional renal impairment unless the obstruction is relieved. The clinical picture may be that of an ill neonate with nonspecific signs and symptoms of infection and renal impairment. Sometimes these features are overshadowed by marked abdominal distension associated with bilateral hydronephrosis, megacystis or urinary ascites (Figure 87). Although the urinary stream may be dribbling, normal micturition does not exclude the diagnosis.

The immediate management is that of fluid, electrolyte and acid–base correction and the use of appropriate antibiotics for the treatment of urinary infection. The valves do not normally obstruct the retrograde passage of a catheter through the urethra for the purpose of a cysto-urethrography (Figure 88), and the valves and their obstructive effects on the bladder may also be visualized by cysto-urethroscopy. Generally these procedures

Figure 86. *Bilateral hydronephrosis and dilated ureters demonstrated by retrograde pyelography. Note extensive clubbing of the renal calyces on the left.*

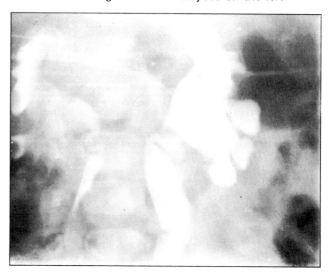

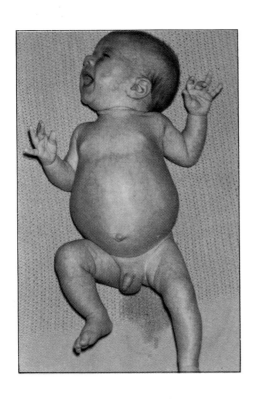

Figure 87. *Marked abdominal distension in association with bilateral hydronephrosis and urinary ascites in a neonate with posterior urethral valves. The stain on the blanket indicates that urinary obstruction was not complete.*

should be immediately followed by operative intervention such as diathermy to the valves via a perineal approach. Occasionally the baby is so ill that definitive surgery has to be delayed and bilateral cutaneous ureterostomies are

Figure 88. *Cysto-urethrogram in a neonate with posterior urethral valves. The dilated proximal urethra is shown inferiorly. There is reflux of dye into a dilated ureter (arrowed).*

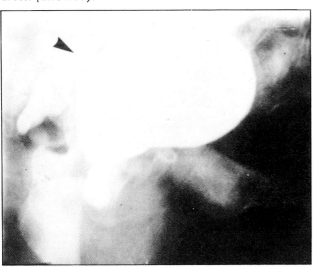

performed to allow urinary drainage and prevent progressive renal damage (Figure 89).

Urinary Tract Infection

Estimates of the incidence of urinary tract infection (UTI) in the neonate range from 0.1 per cent (O'Brien *et al.* 1968) to 1 per cent (Shannon 1970). In contrast to school children and adults, the condition is more common in males and ascending infection is much less common than blood-borne infection. The usual organism is *Escherichia coli*. A high index of suspicion is required for diagnosis because the signs and symptoms are generally nonspecific (Table 44).

Diagnosis

The diagnosis can only be made by urine culture. The problem is to obtain a urine specimen without contamination by organisms that have been introduced into the urine after it has left the bladder. It is usually possible, with patience, to catch a freshly voided specimen in a sterile container. Less satisfactory is the application of an adhesive sterile urine bag. Whichever method is used, significant growth is indicated by the presence of more than 100,000 organisms per ml on a bacterial colony count. However 'significant growth' does not necessarily

Figure 89. *Bilateral ureterostomies in an ill neonate with posterior urethral valves.*

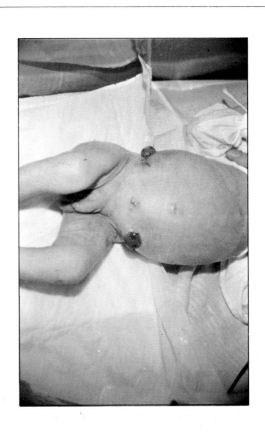

mean 'significant infection' and the diagnosis should always be confirmed by culture of urine obtained by suprapubic aspiration (SPA) (Figure 90). Any growth obtained from an SPA specimen indicates the presence of UTI. When several freshly voided urine specimens contain less than 100,000 organisms per ml, UTI should be excluded by culture of an SPA specimen, whereas if there is no growth, SPA is unnecessary. In many cases urine culture is performed as part of an 'infection screen' in an obviously unwell baby and antibiotics commenced before the results of the various cultures are known. Here the initial urine specimen should be obtained by SPA. However urine is obtained, it should be transported to the bacteriology department without delay.

Management

Persistent infection, particularly in the presence of vesico-ureteric reflux, may lead to renal scarring and impaired renal growth (Smellie and Normand 1968; Rolleston *et al.* 1974). Although details of management may vary, the general aim is the rapid eradication of the infection with the appropriate antibiotic (e.g. gentamycin, ampicillin) followed by a programme of surveillance to detect any recurrence during infancy, radiographic studies to detect abnormalities of the renal tract and, when indicated, serial tests of renal function. After the initial course of antibiotics for two weeks, the urine should be recultured one to two weeks after cessation of therapy and at monthly intervals for at least six months depending on progress. The intravenous pyelogram and micturating cystogram should be performed after the urine has been sterile for several weeks. Vesico-ureteric reflux may be a relatively common occurrence during acute UTI, but persistence of reflux is always abnormal. Recurrence of UTI or its association with radiographic abnormalities is an indication for prophylactic antibiotics. A paediatric surgeon should be involved in surveillance as persistence of infection is often an indication for surgical correction of abnormalities such as vesico-ureteric reflux.

Ambiguous Genitalia

Sexual differentiation of the human fetus is summarized in Figure 91. The presence of ambiguous genitalia is the commonest manifestation of intersex in the neonatal period. Occasionally intersex is manifest in the neonate by the presence of a palpable labial or inguinal gonad (testis) in an apparently normal female. Neonates with ambiguous genitalia may be classified for simplicity into three groups:

1. Female pseudohermaphrodites
2. Male pseudohermaphrodites
3. Those of either sex with abnormalities of gonadal differentiation

Female Pseudohermaphrodites

These have a normal female karyotype (XX), normal internal genitalia and varying degrees of masculinization of the external genitalia (Figure 92). The most common cause is congenital adrenal hyperplasia (CAH), an inborn error of metabolism inherited as an autosomal recessive which leads to a defect in cortisol synthesis in the adrenal gland. Production of adrenocorticotrophin is increased, and adrenal hyperplasia and often a near normal plasma cortisol level are achieved at the cost of an increase in the concentration of androgenic cortisol precursors which cause masculinization of the female external genitalia. Many enzyme defects have been described, but in 90 per cent of cases the enzyme 21-hydroxylase is deficient (Figure 93). Thirty to fifty per cent of these patients cannot synthesize adequate amounts of aldosterone and develop hyponatraemia and hyperkalaemia in association with vomiting and diarrhoea, usually during the second week of life.

Female pseudohermaphroditism may also be caused by the transplacental passage of steroids with androgenic activity. The most common offenders in the 1950s were orally administered synthetic progestogens, but the compounds more recently available have a safer record. Rarely an androgen-secreting maternal tumour causes virilization of a female fetus.

Male Pseudohermaphrodites

These have a normal male karyotype (XY), absence of fallopian tubes and uterus, varying degrees of wolffian duct differentiation, and incomplete masculinization of the external genitalia (Figure 94). The situation may arise from an enzyme defect, causing impaired testosterone synthesis, or a defect in the peripheral action of testosterone. At least five enzyme defects causing impaired synthesis of testosterone have been described. It should be remembered that testosterone synthesis

Figure 90. *Suprapubic aspiration of urine. A wide area of skin over the lower anterior abdominal wall is cleansed with alcohol. A No. 21 sterile disposable needle attached to a 10 ml syringe is used to puncture the skin 1.5 to 2 cm above the pubic symphysis. The needle is advanced towards the fundus, angled 30 degrees from the perpendicular, maintaining a little suction on the syringe. It should not be necessary to introduce the needle to a depth greater than 2.5 cm.*

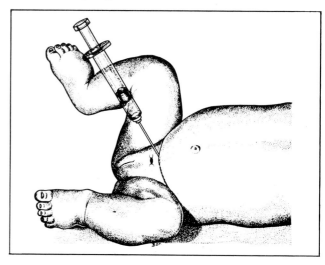

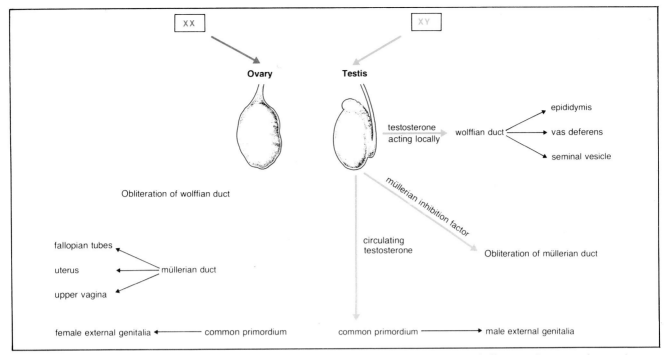

Figure 91. *Sexual differentiation of the human fetus. Note that the sex chromosomes influence the type of gonad formed, and that in the absence of a fetal testis the wolffian duct disappears, the mullerian duct develops into female internal genitalia and female external genitalia develop.*

occurs in the fetal adrenal glands as well as in the testes and certain defects lead to impaired cortisol and testosterone production. These are really examples of CAH associated with incomplete masculinization of male fetuses; moreover salt loss is always present in one form, 3β-hydroxysteroid dehydrogenase deficiency.

The testicular feminization syndrome results from a complete defect in the peripheral action of testosterone, and affected patients have fairly normal testes with male-differentiated internal genital structures, absent uterus, but normal female external genitalia. These patients usually go unrecognized in the neonatal period, although sometimes the testes may be palpated within the labia or pubis or later found during a herniorrhaphy operation. Partial forms of this syndrome occur associated with varying degrees of incomplete masculinization of the external genitalia. The condition is inherited as an X-linked disorder or as an autosomal recessive limited to males.

Abnormalities of Gonadal Differentiation

True hermaphrodites possess both ovarian and testicular tissue and the majority have a normal female karyotype. There is usually a vas deferens on the side of the testis, whereas the ovary is accompanied by a fallopian tube and usually some degree of uterine development. The external genitalia generally appear masculine with hypospadias, bifid scrotum and bilateral cryptorchism. Mixed gonadal dysgenesis is usually associated with mosaicism of the sex chromosomes, the most common being 45XO/46XY. There is usually unilateral testicular development with either a fibrous streak or absent gonadal tissue on the opposite side. The external genitalia vary in appearance from predominantly male with hypospadias and unilateral cryptorchism, to a female appearance with a prominent clitoris and posterior labial fusion.

Management of the Neonate with Ambiguous Genitalia

The parents should be informed that their baby's sex is not certain and that within four weeks (usually much sooner) the appropriate sex will be established after some investigations. Never hazard a guess about sex identity to placate the parents. In the author's experience

Figure 92. *Female pseudohermaphroditism associated with congenital adrenal hyperplasia. The enlarged clitoris is demonstrated.*

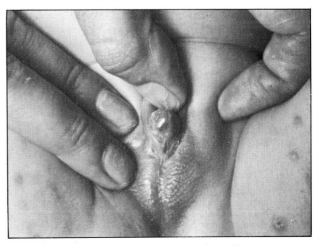

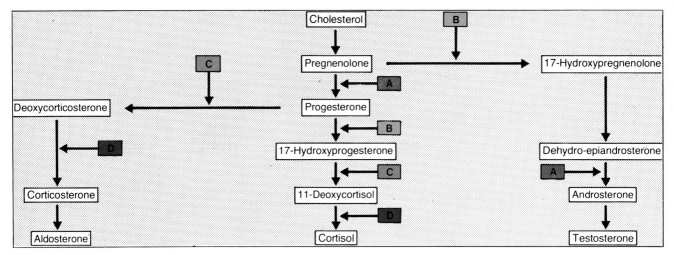

Figure 93. *Metabolic pathways in the production of cortisol, aldosterone and testosterone, showing some of the enzymes involved. A =3ß-hydroxysteroid dehydrogenase; B =17-hydroxylase; C =21-hydroxylase; D =11-hydroxylase.*

the two questions that immediately pre-occupy parents are:

1. "If it's a girl will she be hairy?"
2. "If it's a boy will he be 'queer'?"

A firm "No" should be given to both these questions. It is usually the mother who wants to know the likelihood of a female baby being able to conceive in later years, and further discussion on this aspect should await a definite diagnosis being established. It is helpful to nurse the mother in a single room, preferably in the special care baby unit. It is less easy to shield the mother from numerous relatives and in this respect the baby's father and maternal grandmother can play an important role once the doctor has given them a simple account of the clinical problem and how it is going to be managed. Parents sometimes find it helpful to name the baby early on, chosing from names that are applicable to either sex, although this approach should come from them and not be suggested by the doctor.

A family history and details of drug ingestion during pregnancy should always be sought. The range of possible investigations includes sex chromosome determination, the assay of certain hormones and their precursors in urine and blood, plasma electrolyte determination, radiographic investigation of the genital tract and explorative laparotomy. However, most neonates with ambiguous genitalia are females with CAH due to 21-hydroxylase deficiency and resort to radiography or laparotomy is rarely necessary. There is a real risk of a salt-losing crisis in these patients and therefore close clinical surveillance and frequent monitoring of plasma sodium and potassium levels are necessary in all patients with ambiguous genitalia until the correct diagnosis is established. A 24-hour urinary 17-ketosteroid level of less than 1.0 mg by the end of the second week of life excludes this form of CAH in the absence of prior treatment by glucocorticoids, and detectable quantities of pregnane-

triol in urine or plasma after the first week are virtually diagnostic. The immediate treatment of a neonate with a salt-losing crisis is outlined in Table 45.

Female pseudohermaphrodites are reared as females and require life-long therapy with cortisone acetate. Reproduction is possible. Others are generally reared according to the anatomy of the external genitalia and the decision should always be taken in liaison with the paediatric surgeon, who will subsequently perform reconstructive surgery and be involved in the long-term follow-up of the patient.

Miscellaneous Genital Abnormalities

Cryptorchism

Two to three per cent of term newborn males have unilateral or bilateral cryptorchism and the incidence increases with decreasing gestational age. About 80 per cent of testes not palpable at birth are present in the scrotum by one year of age. However, two important implications of cryptorchism in the neonate are:

1. An inguinal hernia is present in up to 10 per cent of cases and this may require treatment in the first few months of life.

2. When bilateral, or occurring in association with hypospadias, cryptorchism may be a manifestation of intersex.

Hydrocele

A hydrocele manifests as a cystic transilluminable scrotal swelling which is often bilateral. It is caused by persistence of the processus vaginalis allowing peritoneal fluid to accumulate in the tunica vaginalis. Usually the processus vaginalis becomes obliterated spontaneously and the hydrocele reabsorbs during infancy. However a hydrocele is often associated with an inguinal hernia and in this case the hernia should be repaired at the earliest convenience of the family.

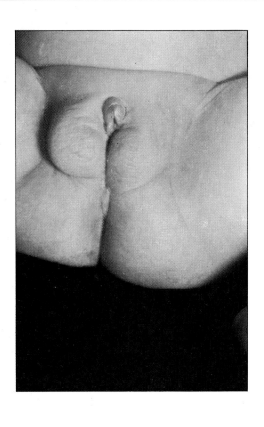

Figure 94. *Male pseudohermaphroditism caused by an incomplete form of testicular feminization syndrome. Testes are present in the unfused scrotum and the phallus is underdeveloped.*

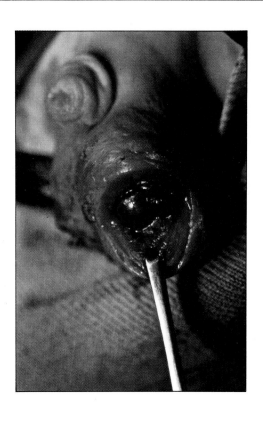

Figure 95. *Torsion of the testis. An infarcted testis shown at operation through a scrotal incision.*

Table 45. Immediate treatment of salt-losing crisis in congenital adrenal hyperplasia.

0.9 per cent saline in 5 per cent dextrose (120–150 ml/kg) intravenously until the baby is rehydrated and vomiting has ceased (usually 24–48 hours).

1 mg aldosterone injection (0.5 mg/ml) intravenously.

4–8 g sodium chloride added to feeds when vomiting has ceased.

In severely shocked babies, 50–100 mg hydrocortisone intravenously followed by 25 mg six hourly.

Testicular Torsion

An oedematous, firm and discoloured scrotum is occasionally present at birth in association with prenatal torsion of a testis. There are surprisingly few systemic manifestations, and the baby generally appears free of pain. At operation through a scrotal incision, the tunica vaginalis and contents are usually found to be infarcted (Figure 95). The torsion is untwisted and unless there is actual sloughing of testicular tissue, the organ is not removed because functional interstitial cells may survive in spite of the ischaemia. The opposite testis is secured by suturing the tunica albuginea to the dartos muscle.

Hydrocolpos

An occluding vaginal membrane may be present at the level of the introitus or higher, causing secretions to accumulate in the vagina. Other abnormalities of the genitourinary tract, lower bowel and lumbosacral spine frequently coexist. The presenting feature is a lower abdominal swelling due to the distended vagina. A bulging membrane may be visible at the vulva. Associated features include swelling of the lower limbs as a result of impaired venous return, and urinary retention. Low membranes may be directly incised at the introitus, whereas an abdominal approach is preferred for high vaginal membranes.

References

Johnston, J. H., *Neonatal Surgery* (Ed. Rickham, P. P. and Johnston, J. H.), page 603, Butterworths, London, 1970.

O'Brien, N. G., Carroll, R., Donovan, D. E. and Dundon, S. P., *J. Irish Med. Ass.,* 1968, **61**, 267.

Rolleston, G. L., Shannon, F. T. and Utley, W. L. F., *Brit. Med. J.,* 1974, **1**, 460.

Shannon, F. T., *Pediat. Clin. N. Amer.,* 1970, **18**, 512.

Smellie, J. C. and Normand, I. C. S., *Urinary Tract Infection* (Ed. O'Grady, F. and Brumfitt, W.), page 123, Oxford University Press, Oxford and London, 1968.

Williams, D. I., *Congenital Abnormalities in Infancy* (Ed. Norman, A. P.), page 204, Blackwell Scientific Publications, Oxford and Edinburgh, 1971.

12. Metabolic Adaptation to Extrauterine Life

 METABOLISM in the fetus is powerfully influenced by an inter-relationship between maternal and feto-placental metabolism. The measurement of plasma concentrations of biochemicals in the immediate newborn period is a crude guide to metabolic function. However, the fact that well defined sequential changes do occur with respect to many biochemicals suggests a metabolic adaptation to extrauterine life. This chapter draws attention to several examples of suboptimal metabolic adaptation. Often the problem is of a transient nature. Occasionally permanent metabolic derangements, for example, familial disorders of intermediary metabolism, are revealed in the neonatal period. The endocrine system influences numerous metabolic processes; certain disorders of adrenal gland function have been discussed in relation to ambiguous genitalia in Chapter 11. Congenital hypothyroidism and thyrotoxicosis will be discussed here because of their important therapeutic implications.

Hypoglycaemia

Carbohydrate is the principal source of energy for the fetus, and glucose is continuously transferred from the maternal circulation across the placenta down a concentration gradient. Fetal blood glucose levels are generally 50 to 80 per cent of maternal levels. Insulin is present in the fetal pancreas from the eleventh week and the concentration increases with gestational age (Steinke and Driscoll 1965). However, glucose loads presented to the fetus from 11 to 20 weeks do not cause additional insulin secretion, and even at term the fetal insulin response to a glucose load given to the mother is small and sluggish (Adam et al. 1969; Milner and Hales 1965). The placenta is more or less impermeable to insulin. During labour and immediately after birth, fetal glycogen stores in the liver and heart are an immediately available source of energy essential to survival. Hepatic glycogen stores are soon depleted by initial glycogenolysis, and a rapid fall in the blood glucose concentration during the first two hours of life is a normal occurrence. During the course of two or three days there is a switch over to the use of fat as a source of energy, and soon after birth plasma free fatty acid levels increase and there is a fall in the respiratory quotient. There is also increasing gluconeogenesis from amino acids.

The brain essentially requires glucose for metabolism,

and the extent to which other substances such as ketone bodies act as a source of energy for the brain of a neonate is uncertain. Hypoglycaemia exists whenever available glucose fails to meet the metabolic requirements of brain cells. One arbitrary definition of neonatal hypoglycaemia is a blood glucose concentration less than 30 mg per cent (1.66 mmol/l) in a baby who weighs more than 2.5 kg, and a level less than 20 mg per cent (1.11 mmol/l) in a baby under 2.5 kg. This definition does not mean that any level of blood glucose above the diagnostic value is always safe. It is merely a working definition that hopefully allows the clinician to detect on the basis of a biochemical measurement most babies in whom there is failure or *impending failure* of glucose to meet the metabolic requirements of brain cells.

Hypoglycaemia may be symptomatic or asymptomatic and come to light when blood glucose measurements are routinely performed in babies known to be at risk. There are no specific signs or symptoms of hypoglycaemia but the clinical features shown in Table 46 have been reported in association with abnormally low blood glucose levels and have abated when normoglycaemia was achieved with treatment. The situations in which hypoglycaemia is prone to occur are shown in Table 47, and three of these of special importance are discussed below. The precise pathogenesis of hypoglycaemia in various conditions is usually imperfectly understood. It may result whenever there is insufficient peripheral release of glucose or increased peripheral uptake and utilization. In some circumstances both factors operate. The complexity of the problem results from the fact that the release and uptake of glucose in different tissues are controlled by many inter-related mechanisms.

Table 46. Signs and symptoms associated with hypoglycaemia.

Apathy and hypotonia
Refusal to feed
Cyanosis
Apnoeic attacks
Tremulous or jittery movements
Convulsions
Eye rolling
Temperature instability

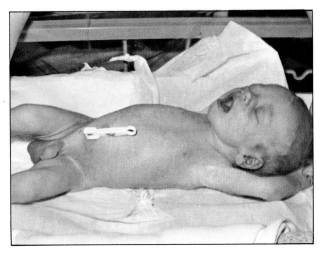

Figure 96. *Small for dates neonates. Note the mature, well-formed ears and genitalia of this baby who was born at term and suffered from intrauterine malnutrition.*

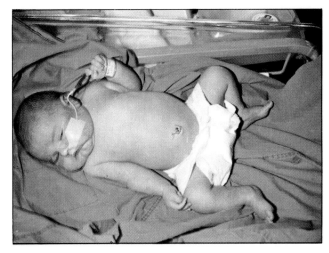

Figure 97. *Infant of a diabetic mother. The baby is large for dates and the face has a cherubic appearance. Feeding by nasogastric tube was necessary to ensure an adequate milk intake in the presence of early hypoglycaemia.*

Predisposing Factors

Small for dates babies. The onset of signs and symptoms is often delayed until 24 to 72 hours after delivery or even longer, and treatment may have to be continued for a week or more until satisfactory blood glucose levels are achieved (see 'Management' below). Small for dates (SFD) babies (Figure 96) are prone to perinatal asphyxia, making them particularly vulnerable to severe hypoglycaemia. One problem is that signs and symptoms may be wholly attributed to an episode of preceding asphyxia, and treatable hypoglycaemia neglected. Several mechanisms probably contribute to the hypoglycaemia in SFD babies, including insufficient stores of liver glycogen, delay in the development of hepatic gluconeogenesis (Haymond *et al.* 1974), relative hyperinsulinaemia and deficient catecholamine secretion. Small for dates babies are a heterogeneous group: some are the products of multiple pregnancy, others have suffered *in utero* from a maternal complication of pregnancy, and there are those whose smallness is genetically determined. It is unlikely that the pathogenesis of hypoglycaemia is the same in all SFD babies.

Babies of diabetic mothers. Hypoglycaemia occurs in about 50 per cent of all babies delivered of diabetic mothers (Wald 1973). The onset is usually within six hours of birth, and more than 90 per cent of affected babies are asymptomatic. The aetiology is hypertrophy and hyperplasia of the islets of Langerhans caused by intermittent fetal hyperglycaemia. Hyperinsulinaemia occurs *in utero* and promotes lipogenesis and fetal growth. This is partly responsible for the characteristic appearance of the baby (Figure 97). After birth, when the maternal supply of glucose is cut off, relative hyperinsulinaemia persists and the blood glucose concentration falls precipitously. It must be remembered that transient hypoglycaemia is also a feature of babies born to mothers

whose diabetes is controlled by diet alone, and serious intractable hypoglycaemia may occur when the mother has been treated with oral sulphonylureas. These insulinotropic drugs are only slowly degraded by the neonate.

Haemolytic disease of the newborn. Hyperplasia of the islets of Langerhans and hyperinsulinaemia occur in severe haemolytic disease, most commonly Rhesus incompatibility. Hypoglycaemia during the first day of life is a common finding in those born with profound anaemia and hepatosplenomegaly, and should not be overlooked during resuscitation. The cause of the pancreatic hyperplasia is not clear. One theory is that it occurs as a response to increased insulin destruction either by the hypertrophied placenta or by glutathione which accumulates in the blood as a result of massive haemolysis (Schiff and Lowy 1970; Steinke *et al.* 1967). Hypoglycaemia is also prone to occur following exchange

Table 47. Situations in which hypoglycaemia is prone to occur.

Small for dates babies
Very low birth weight (< 1.5 kg)
Babies of diabetic mothers
Haemolytic disease of the newborn
After exchange transfusion with ACD blood
Idiopathic respiratory distress syndrome
Perinatal asphyxia
Hypothermia
Severe sepsis
Less common:
    Inborn errors of metabolism
    Beckwith's syndrome (visceromegaly, large tongue, exomphalos)
    Adrenal insufficiency
    Pancreatic islet cell tumour

Table 48. Hypoglycaemia: monitoring with Dextrostix and criteria for conservative management.

Monitor the following babies:

Small for dates	6 hourly for 72 hours, then daily until 7 days
Maternal diabetes	4, 8, 12, 24 hours
Very low birthweight (< 1.5 kg)	12, 24, 48, 72 hours
Those suffering from:	
perinatal asphyxia	Soon after resuscitation, 2, 6, 12 hours
haemolytic disease	6 hourly for first day: 1, 3, 6 hours after exchange transfusion
idiopathic respiratory distress	Whenever blood gas measurements made
hypothermia	Several times until body temperature > 36°C
severe sepsis	8 hourly

Criteria for conservative management:

Absence of signs or symptoms attributable to hypoglycaemia
Normal tolerance to oral feeds
   Birth weight > 1.5 kg
   Not small for dates
   Trend towards increasing blood glucose levels in 6 to 12 hours

---

transfusion because the extra glucose load presented to the baby in the form of acid–citrate–dextrose preserved blood, stimulates insulin secretion.

Management

Certain babies (see Table 48) should be screened for hypoglycaemia using the Dextrostix method and the results read with the aid of a reflectance meter (Ames Ltd). Values less than 20 mg per cent (1.11 mmol/l) should be confirmed by the laboratory. It may be argued that all babies with abnormally low levels ought to have normoglycaemia rapidly restored by intravenous dextrose therapy. This is unnecessary because, with the prompt institution of milk feeds, the blood glucose concentration increases in many neonates who have asymptomatic hypoglycaemia soon after birth. There is little point in feeding such babies orally with a 10 per cent dextrose solution, which is prone to cause diarrhoea by its osmotic effect. Milk feeding and vigilance is an acceptable form of management providing the criteria shown in Table 48 are adhered to. Intravenous dextrose therapy is mandatory if any of these criteria is not obtained. A guide to intravenous therapy is presented in Table 49. Critical attention to detail is essential. The infusion site must be inspected at frequent intervals because 'resistant hypoglycaemia' may indicate that the infusion has become extravascular. The blood glucose concentration should be monitored hourly for the first six hours and then four-hourly. The repeated administration of concentrated solutions of dextrose in bolus form should be avoided because hyperinsulinaemia and rebound hypoglycaemia are liable to occur. The unnecessary use of rapid infusion rates, or 15 per cent dextrose when 10 per cent dextrose would suffice, may cause glycosuria and polyuria with secondary electrolyte disturbances

Prognosis

The incidence of severe neurological sequelae such as mental retardation, fits and cerebral palsy following inadequately treated symptomatic hypoglycaemia is very high (perhaps 30 to 50 per cent), whereas the prognosis is very much better for properly treated symptomatic neonates. Those with asymptomatic hypoglycaemia, such as babies of diabetic mothers, generally fare well.

Hypocalcaemia

Calcium is actively transported across the placenta to the fetus, and at birth the serum calcium concentration of the baby is about 1.0 mg per cent (0.25 mmol/l) greater than the maternal level. Soon after birth the serum calcium concentration in the baby falls, reaching a mean value of

---

Table 49. Guide to intravenous therapy for hypoglycaemia.

INITIAL INJECTION (if symptoms present):
5 ml 20 per cent dextrose via a peripheral vein, *always followed by:*

MAINTENANCE THERAPY:
70 to 90 ml/kg/24 hours of 10 per cent dextrose plus oral feeds (if tolerated):
60 to 80 ml/kg/24 hours of milk

IF NORMOGLYCAEMIA NOT MAINTAINED:
1. Check infusion site.
2. Increase rate of infusion up to 150 ml/kg/24 hours, and reduce oral feeds accordingly or change infusion to 15 per cent dextrose.
3. Check Dextrostix: avoid hyperglycaemia and glycosuria.

IF NORMOGLYCAEMIA STILL NOT MAINTAINED:
1. Check infusion site.
2. Add hydrocortisone 5 mg/kg to the infusion fluid every 12 hours or add ACTH 4 units/kg every 12 hours.
3. In the light of subsequent progress it may be necessary to consider unusual causes of hypoglycaemia, e.g. inborn metabolic error, islet cell tumour etc.

N.B. A constant infusion pump rather than a manually operated i.v. line should be used.

about 7.5 mg per cent (1.88 mmol/l) on the second day. Thereafter the level rises towards adult values during the next two to three days. Some babies, particularly those ingesting relatively large quantities of phosphate in their milk, experience a second fall in the serum calcium level at five to seven days.

Hypocalcaemia may be arbitrarily defined as a serum calcium concentration less than 7.5 mg per cent (1.85 mmol/l). However the total serum calcium, which is usually measured, does not accurately reflect the concentration of ionized calcium which is of physiological importance.

Clinical Syndromes

Symptoms attributed to hypocalcaemia are nonspecific and include twitching, 'jitteryness', fits, cyanotic and apnoeic attacks and vomiting. The elicitation of Chvostek's sign is of little help in the diagnosis as it is present in many normal neonates. A minority of neonates with symptomatic hypocalcaemia exhibit Trousseau's sign. There are two clinical syndromes of hypocalcaemia from a practical viewpoint:

Early onset hypocalcaemia. This occurs during the first 48 hours of life in certain vulnerable babies (Table 50), and is an exaggeration of the normal fall in serum calcium that occurs soon after birth. Many aetiological factors have been proposed, including transient parathyroid gland suppression, poor calcium intake, reduced ionic dissociation of calcium as a result of bicarbonate administration, and hyperphosphataemia, perhaps as a response to increased maternal or fetal adrenocortical gland secretion or as a result of a catabolic state in babies who have suffered a traumatic labour and delivery or whose caloric intake is poor. However, only a minority of babies with early onset hypocalcaemia are hyperphosphataemic. Calcitonin, a hormone with an antiosteolytic and hypocalcaemic action, is released in response to anoxia and may play a role in the aetiology. Early onset hypocalcaemia occurs in a group of babies who often manifest abnormal clinical signs and symptoms for other reasons. It is not uncommon for hypoglycaemia and hypocalcaemia to coexist in such babies.

Classical neonatal tetany. The onset is typically between five and seven days and symptoms may last from several days to two weeks. The condition is virtually confined to babies fed with cow's milk preparations. Although the calcium content of cow's milk is greater than human milk, the calcium to phosphate ratio is considerably lower. The kidneys are presented with a relatively high phosphate load which cannot be adequately excreted because of transient parathyroid suppression and possibly impaired renal responsiveness to parathyroid hormone. A fall in the serum calcium level occurs, presumably because a hyperphosphataemic state does not favour osteolysis and calcium release from bone. It is likely that the incidence of neonatal tetany has fallen with the introduction of humanized milk preparations with a smaller phosphate content.

Table 50. Factors associated with neonatal hypocalcaemia.

Early onset:
Prematurity
Birth trauma
Perinatal asphyxia
Maternal diabetes mellitus
Use of i.v. bicarbonate
Idiopathic respiratory distress syndrome

Classical neonatal tetany:
Peak incidence 5 to 7 days
Use of cow's milk formulae with low Ca:PO$_4$ ratio
Serum phosphate elevated

Other types of hypocalcaemia:
During exchange transfusion with citrated blood
Maternal hyperparathyroidism
Maternal osteomalacia
Di George's syndrome
Congenital hypoparathyroidism

Other Hypocalcaemic Syndromes

These are shown in Table 50 and, with the exception of hypocalcaemia associated with exchange transfusion, are relatively rare. The ionized serum calcium concentration falls abruptly during exchange transfusion with citrated blood. The traditional administration of 1 ml of 10 per cent calcium gluconate after each 100 ml of blood exchanged merely causes a transient increase in ionized calcium immediately after the dose is given (Maisels *et al.* 1974). Occasionally severe tetany, early in onset and prolonged, is the first clue to the presence of a maternal parathyroid adenoma.

The Di George syndrome consists of absence of parathyroid and thymic tissue with facial arch abnormalities (e.g. ears, palate). Affected patients are vulnerable to sepsis because of impaired cell-mediated immunity, and hypocalcaemia is commonly of early onset. True congenital hypoparathyroidism as opposed to a transient form has been described in neonates and responds to treatment with parathyroid hormone.

Treatment

Parenteral therapy carries the hazards of bradycardia and cardiac arrest if the injection is given too rapidly. Calcium solutions are irritants, and leakage outside the vein is prone to occur when the baby is irritable or jittery during the injection. It is probably preferable to treat fits or twitching with intramuscular phenobarbitone. Although some paediatricians recommend giving parenteral calcium as a diagnostic test in babies with fits, it should be remembered that calcium often acts in a nonspecific way and may even control fits associated with hypoglycaemia.

When frequent apnoeic attacks occur in association with hypocalcaemia (a not uncommon finding in ill babies with idiopathic respiratory distress syndrome), it is reasonable to use parenteral calcium. In the author's experience, however, correction of the serum calcium level in this situation rarely influences the course of the

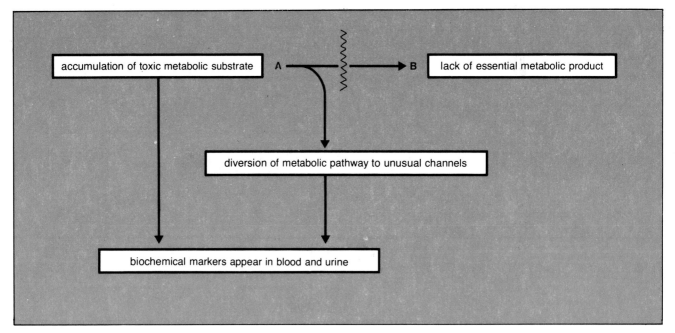

Figure 98. *Disorders of intermediary metabolism. Sequence of events that occurs when substance A (e.g. an amino acid) cannot be converted to substance B because of a genetically determined lack of specific enzyme.*

apnoeic attacks. A suitable parenteral dose is 1 to 2 ml/kg of 10 per cent calcium gluconate given through an established intravenous line at a rate no faster than 1 ml per minute. The electrocardiogram should be monitored during the injection, which should be terminated if bradycardia occurs. Suitable oral regimens are 2 to 3 g per day of calcium lactate solution (13 per cent calcium) or 2 to 4 g per day of calcium gluconate (9 per cent calcium) in four to six divided doses. Oral therapy should be continued for two to three days after the serum calcium level has returned to normal. Milk given to hypocalcaemic babies should have a relatively low phosphate content—ideally breast milk, or, failing this, one of the 'humanized' milk preparations.

Prognosis

The prognosis in 'classical' neonatal tetany is excellent. However, when symptoms occur associated with hypocalcaemia of early onset, the prognosis is influenced by the presence of complicating factors such as birth asphyxia and trauma, prematurity *per se,* idiopathic respiratory distress syndrome, etc.

Hypomagnesaemia

This has been observed in association with hypocalcaemia irrespective of the underlying cause. In addition it has been described secondary to maternal magnesium deficiency, and in infants with magnesium malabsorption. Signs and symptoms of hypomagnesaemia are indistinguishable from those of hypocalcaemia, although bilateral pitting oedema of the feet was a feature of certain babies with neonatal tetany who had associated hypomagnesaemia (Chiswick 1971).

The normal range of serum magnesium in neonates is influenced by methodology but generally levels less than 1.5 mg per cent are considered to be abnormally low. One suggested form of therapy is magnesium sulphate (0.2 ml of 50 per cent solution) given intramuscularly and repeated twelve hours later if necessary. When hypocalcaemia and hypomagnesaemia coexist it is sometimes observed that in spite of calcium supplements the serum calcium does not increase until the hypomagnesaemia has been corrected.

Inherited Metabolic Abnormalities

Severe constraints may be put upon metabolic functions by virtue of genetic abnormalities. Individually, inborn errors of metabolism are rare. Their importance is, first, that prompt diagnosis and dietary manipulation may control certain diseases, and, second, their genetic implications, with the possible risk of further offspring being affected. The clinical manifestations of inborn errors of metabolism are protean. Rather than detail individual diseases, the following account outlines certain principles that will help the clinician to decide if an ill neonate could be suffering from an inherited metabolic abnormality. When such a diagnosis is likely the detailed biochemical work-up requires the services of a specialist laboratory and a paediatrician with experience of this group of disorders. There are three main types of inherited metabolic abnormality:

1. Defects of membrane transport affecting the passage of small molecules such as amino acids and sugars from the lumen of the intestine or renal tubule.

2. Abnormal storage of material in the cells of certain

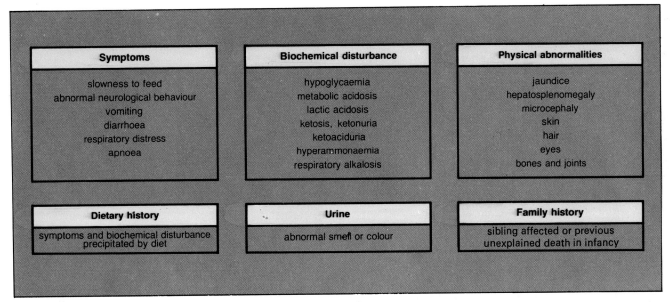

Figure 99. *Clues to the diagnosis of inherited metabolic disorders.*

organs leading to organ enlargement and impairment of function.

3. Deficiency of enzymes of intermediary metabolism (Figure 98).

A combination of some of the factors shown in Figure 99 suggests the presence of an inherited metabolic abnormality. The majority are inherited as an autosomal recessive with a recurrence risk of 25 per cent, and a previous unexplained death in early infancy should arouse suspicion. Certain biochemical disturbances are common to many different inherited metabolic disorders, and may be precipitated by milk feeds. Hypoglycaemia that occurs unexpectedly or runs an atypical course should arouse suspicion. The mechanism underlying a metabolic acidosis is often obscure, but contributory factors may include the accumulation of lactic acid or abnormal metabolites that interfere with oxidative catabolism and cause ketoacidaemia. The excretion of ketoacids in the urine (ketoaciduria) occurs in disorders of branch chain amino acid metabolism. Hyperammonaemia is a feature of metabolic disturbances involving the urea cycle and there is usually a positive temporal relationship with protein ingestion. An associated mild respiratory alkalosis sometimes occurs.

An abnormal smell or colour of the urine in an ill neonate may be a clue to the presence of a metabolic disorder, and comments made by the nurses are particularly valuable because they have become accustomed to a wide range of neonatal urine. Storage diseases in particular may be associated with physical abnormalities such as hepatosplenomegaly, skeletal dysplasia and thickening and loss of elasticity of the skin. Abnormalities of the eye involving the cornea, lens or retina also occur in many non-storage metabolic disorders.

Table 51. Preliminary urine tests for metabolic disorders.

Reagent	Method	Interpretation
Acetest tablet	Place drop of urine on the tablet	Purple—ketonuria Red, yellow—proprionicaciduria —methylmalonicaciduria
Clinitest tablet Clinistix	Follow instructions supplied with reagent	Positive Clinitest—reducing substance Positive Clinistix—glucose
Ferric chloride, 10 per cent (w/v) in 0.25 N HCl	Add reagent dropwise to 1 ml of urine. Observe colour at 1 to 3 minutes	Blue–green—phenylketonuria Grey–green—histidinaemia Blue, yellow, blue–green— ketoaciduria Yellow—hyperalininaemia Brown—ketonuria
Saturated solution of 2,4 DNP hydrazine in HCl	Mix equal volumes of urine and reagent. Observe at 1 minute	Yellow or red precipitate— ketoaciduria

Sodium cyanide, 5 per cent (w/v)
in water. Sodium nitroprusside
(freshly made solution containing
a few crystals in water)
	Mix equal volumes of urine and
	sodium cyanide solution and leave
	for 10 minutes. Add 3 to 4 drops
	of nitroprusside reagent
		Magenta—cystinuria
		        —homocystinuria
		        —generalized aminoaciduria

Several simple biochemical tests on blood or urine are helpful when a metabolic disorder is suspected (Table 51). In a seriously ill neonate, the substitution of parenteral 10 per cent dextrose for protein feeding may be a life-saving measure prior to liaison with the specialist laboratory for definitive investigation.

Abnormalities of Thyroid Function

The fetal pituitary–thyroid axis functions autonomously, and placental transfer of thyroid stimulating hormone (TSH), triiodothyronine (T_3) and thyroxine (T_4), does not occur to a significant degree. There is a marked increase in serum TSH concentration during the first two hours of life and this is paralleled by a rise in the T_3 level. The serum concentration of both hormones declines to normal levels by 48 hours. Serum T_4 concentration increases more slowly than T_3 after birth, and a peak value is achieved at about 24 hours.

Congenital Hypothyroidism

The causes are shown in Table 52. Agenesis or dysgenesis of the thyroid gland is the most common cause of congenital hypothyroidism in the UK. Babies with residual thyroid tissue in the normal or ectopic site (e.g. lingual) may not develop clinical features until later in infancy. Others with more severe lack of thyroid hormone *in utero* have suggestive signs and symptoms early on (see Figure 100 and Table 53). A high index of suspicion is required for prompt diagnosis, so that replacement therapy can be commenced as soon as possible. The final outcome in terms of growth and mental development is influenced by the duration of thyroid insufficiency.

Table 52. Some causes of congenital hypothyroidism.

Agenesis or dysgenesis of the thyroid gland
Endemic goitrous hypothyroidism
Maternally administered antithyroid drugs (e.g. iodides, thiourea derivatives)
Inborn errors of thyroxine synthesis
Defect of thyroglobulin
End-organ unresponsiveness to thyroid hormone
Unresponsiveness of thyroid to TSH

Table 53. Signs and symptoms of congenital hypothyroidism.

Prolonged neonatal jaundice
Lethargy and slowness to feed
Respiratory difficulty and intermittent cyanosis
Coarse facial appearance, flattened nasal bridge, enlarged tongue.
Hoarse cry
Constipation
Protuberant abdomen and umbilical hernia
Bradycardia
Hypothermia

Note that signs in the neonatal period are often absent or consist only of prolonged neonatal jaundice, lethargy and slowness to feed.

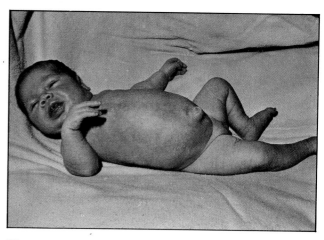

Figure 100. *Congenital hypothyroidism. This lethargic baby has slight abdominal distension and a small umbilical hernia. Note the protuberant tongue.*

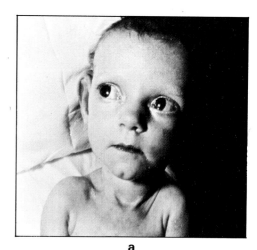

a

Figure 101. *Neonatal thyrotoxicosis.* **a)** *This hyperactive neonate suffered considerable weight loss in spite of a voracious appetite. Note the prominent eyes.* **b)** *Enlargement of the thyroid gland.*

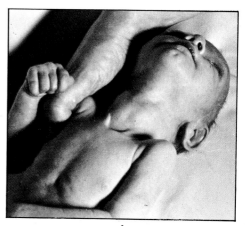

b

The single most helpful laboratory test is the serum TSH concentration, which is raised beyond 48 hours of life in hypothyroidism with a functioning pituitary gland. Each laboratory should determine its own 'normal range' because results vary according to methodology. Treatment is with L-thyroxine 0.05 mg daily, rapidly increasing to 0.1 mg daily. It has been suggested that the smallest dose of thyroxine which maintains the TSH level in the normal range is the optimal dose (Barnes 1975). Treatment is for life, and one situation that sometimes arises is that of the baby who loses the physical stigmata and develops relatively normally on replacement therapy. If such a patient comes under the care of a different practitioner in a new area the original diagnosis may be doubted and therapy stopped. The mother ought to retain a clinical photograph of her baby taken before treatment, illustrating the physical stigmata.

Transient Neonatal Thyrotoxicosis

This serious but self-limiting disorder is liable to occur in babies born to mothers who have active thyrotoxicosis or a past history of the disease. The transplacental passage of long-acting thyroid stimulator (LATS), an immunoglobulin G, may be responsible for neonatal thyrotoxicosis, although cases have been reported in which the transplacental passage of another immunoglobulin, human thyroid stimulating immunoglobulin (HTSI), has been implicated (Mitchell et al. 1976; Nutt et al. 1974). The clinical features may take several days to appear. They include over-activity, ravenous appetite but poor weight gain, diarrhoea, tachycardia, heart failure, proptosis and enlargement of the thyroid gland (Figure 101). Treatment consists of potassium iodide (5 mg, eight-

hourly, orally). Carbimazole (2.5 mg, eight-hourly, orally) may also be necessary. Heart failure may be treated with digoxin. Once the symptoms are under control the drugs may be gradually withdrawn, and treatment is rarely necessary beyond four weeks of age. Recently the β-adrenergic blocking agent propranolol has been introduced as a treatment for neonatal thyrotoxicosis (Pemberton et al. 1974).

References

Adam, P. A. J., Teramo, K., Raiha, N., Gitlin, D. and Schwartz, R., *Diabetes,* 1969, **18**, 409.

Barnes, N. D., *Arch. Dis. Childh.,* 1975, **50**, 497.

Chiswick, M. L., *Brit. Med. J.,* 1971, **3**, 15.

Haymond, M. W., Karl, I. E. and Pagleara, A. S., *New. Engl. J. Med.,* 1974, **291**, 322.

Maisels, M. J., Li, T-K., Piechocki, J. T. and Werthman, M. W., *Pediatrics,* 1974, **53**, 683.

Milner, R. D. G. and Hales, C. N., *Brit. Med. J.,* 1965, **1**, 284.

Mitchell, I., Shenfield, G. and Brash, J., *Arch. Dis. Childh.,* 1976, **51**, 565.

Nutt, J., Clark, F., Welch, R. G. and Hall, R., *Brit. Med. J.,* 1974, **4**, 695.

Pemberton, P. J., McConnell, B. and Shanks, R. G., *Arch. Dis. Childh.,* 1974, **49**, 813.

Schiff, D. and Lowy, C., *Pediat. Res.,* 1970, **4**, 280.

Steinke, J. and Driscoll, S., *Diabetes,* 1965, **14**, 573.

Steinke, J., Gries, F. A. and Driscoll, S., *Blood,* 1967, **30**, 359.

Wald, M. K., *Care of the High Risk Neonate,* page 171 (Eds Klaus, M. H. and Fanaroff, A. A.), W. B. Saunders Co., London, 1973.

Further Reading

Nathanielsz, P. W., *Fetal Endocrinology,* Elsevier-North Holland, The Netherlands, 1976.

13. Modern Concepts in Maternal and Infant Care

Congenital Abnormality

PROBABLY about half of all conceptions are aborted, many at a very early stage of development (Boué *et al.* 1975). Sixty per cent of spontaneous abortions in the first trimester are associated with chromosome abnormalities, trisomy syndromes accounting for 50 per cent of these and Turner's syndrome (45XO) for 20 per cent. It is clear that nature recognizes and deals appropriately with most of her imperfections. However, two to three per cent of newborn babies have a significant abnormality which is immediately apparent on examination or is revealed during the first week of life. The incidence of different types of malformation shown in Table 54 is probably underestimated because of under-reporting. The true incidence of chromosome abnormalities in the newborn, for example, is nearer six per 1,000 when babies born consecutively are studied (Grouchy 1976).

Whereas in the past the birth of a malformed baby was inclined to be surrounded by taboo, today's mother-to-be, even before conception, may express her anxieties about the possibility of giving birth to an abnormal baby. One stimulus for this change in attitude has been the altered pattern of mortality and morbidity in infancy. Twenty-five years ago congenital malformations accounted for 14 per cent of infant deaths in England and Wales, but the corresponding figure in 1974 was 24 per cent. However,

in absolute terms the number of infant deaths from malformations per 1,000 live births has remained relatively constant (about four per 1,000). Other factors responsible for the increase in parental awareness of the risk of congenital malformations include the development of prenatal diagnostic techniques and methods of treating certain congenital abnormalities. These tools have emotive and ethical implications that have been exploited by the popular press and television before the medical profession has had time to learn how to use them most effectively for the benefit of patients. There is no doubt that genetic counselling services and facilities for prenatal diagnosis are now insufficient to meet public demands.

Genetic Counselling

The commonest reasons for parents seeking advice are:

1. The previous birth of an abnormal baby.

2. The presence of an abnormality in one or both parents or in other members of their family.

3. High maternal age.

The term 'genetic counselling' as commonly used is misleading in implying that most congenital abnormalities result from gene or chromosomal defects with a well-defined recurrence risk. In fact this is only the case in a minority of birth defects. Environmental factors combined with genetic factors are responsible for most birth defects and in many cases the risk of a baby having such defects can only be expressed empirically (see below). When assessing the risk of recurrence of an abnormality that has already affected a member of the family, the availability of an accurate description and diagnosis of the condition and a detailed family history powerfully influence the accuracy of any risk estimate. Examples of abnormalities with different modes of inheritance are shown in Table 55. Some clinical implications of different modes of inheritance will be discussed briefly.

Autosomal Dominant

1. Every patient has one affected parent and when a pedigree chart is constructed a 'vertical line' of transmission is apparent.

2. One in two of the offspring of an affected parent has the condition.

Table 54. Incidence (per 1,000 total births) of various types of congenital malformation in England and Wales in 1973.

Congenital malformation	Incidence per 1000 births
Limbs	6.7
CNS	3.7
External genitals	1.7
Cleft lip and/or cleft palate	1.4
Cardiovascular	1.1
Chromosomal	0.8
Intestines	0.7
Ear	0.6
Eye	0.1

Data from Office of Population Censuses and Surveys.

Table 55. Mode of inheritance of certain congenital abnormalities.

Autosomal dominant
    Achondroplasia
    Osteogenesis imperfecta
    Tuberous sclerosis
    Marfan's syndrome
    Myotonia congenita
    Spherocytosis

Autosomal recessive
    Cystic fibrosis
    Disorders of amino acid metabolism
    Galactosaemia
    Adrenogenital syndromes
    Werdnig–Hoffmann disease (infantile onset)
    Tay–Sachs disease
    Sickle cell anaemia
    Thalassaemia

X-linked recessive
    Haemophilia A and B
    Duchenne's muscular dystrophy
    Lowe's syndrome
    Glucose-6-phosphate dehydrogenase deficiency
    Hunter's syndrome
    Nephrogenic diabetes insipidus

X-linked dominant
    Vitamin-D-resistant rickets
    Pseudohypoparathyroidism

3. Normal individuals do not transmit the abnormality to their offspring.

There are pitfalls to tax the counsellor. Certain conditions inherited in this way may only be partially expressed or not expressed at all in a genetically affected (heterozygote) parent. Conditions known to be inherited as an autosomal dominant may occur as a gene mutation in which case neither parent has the harmful gene and both are clinically normal. Nevertheless the affected individual still has a one in two chance of transmitting the harmful mutant gene to his or her offspring.

Autosomal Recessive

1. Affected patients have clinically normal parents (unaffected heterozygotes or carriers).

2. One in four children born to such parents is clinically affected and two in three of the unaffected children receive the causative gene and become carriers.

3. The mode of inheritance is generally only recognized after one or more affected offspring have been born.

4. Clinically affected patients who marry normal individuals (non-carriers) have clinically normal offspring, but one in two receives the causative gene and becomes a carrier.

5. Amongst the parents of those who manifest rare autosomal recessive conditions there is a relatively high incidence of consanguineous marriages.

It is possible to calculate the frequency of carriers of a harmful recessive gene from knowledge of the incidence of the disease. The frequency of carriers is $2pq$, where q^2 is the homozygote frequency (or the incidence of the disease) and $p = 1 - q$ (Hardy–Weinberg principle).

X-Linked Recessive

Clinical abnormality is manifest in the male carrying an abnormal gene on the X chromosome whereas the female carrier is clinically normal.

1. An affected male cannot transmit the disease to his son.

2. All the daughters of an affected male are carriers.

3. A carrier female transmits the disease to half her sons and transmits the carrier state to half her daughters.

Essentially the problem is that of detection of the clinically normal female carrier. An important pitfall is the fact that affected males and carrier females may be mutants and of course the sisters of mutants are not at risk of receiving the abnormal gene. A female is a carrier if:

1. Her father is affected.

2. She has more than one affected son.

3. She has one affected son *and* her maternal uncle or maternal great uncle, or maternal cousin or sister's son is affected.

In a few X-linked recessive conditions it is possible to suspect female carriers with varying degrees of certainty by careful physical examination (e.g. lens opacities in Lowe's syndrome), or by biochemical tests (e.g. raised serum creatine kinase activity in Duchenne-type muscular dystrophy).

X-Linked Dominant

1. An affected male cannot transmit the disease to his son.

2. All his daughters are clinically affected.

3. An affected female transmits the disease to one in two of her children (sons *and* daughters).

Empirical Risks

Congenital malformations often have a familial tendency which is not compatible with any of the well-defined lines of inheritance. Environmental factors probably contribute to their aetiology. Empirical risk estimates are generally based on accumulated data which show the distribution of cases in families and the frequency of occurrence in relatives of index cases.

Prenatal Diagnosis of Congenital Abnormality

Certain abnormalities may be diagnosed or suspected before 20 weeks' gestation, providing an opportunity for termination of pregnancy. Genetic counselling and prenatal diagnosis are complementary services in that counselling usually provides the stimulus for attempting prenatal diagnosis. Diagnostic methods include radiography, ultrasonics and amniocentesis with biochemical or chromosomal analysis of cultured cells shed from the fetus or biochemical examination of cell-free fluid. Generally the most common reasons for diagnostic amniocentesis in this context are for the diagnosis of Down's syndrome (chromosome analysis) and open neural-tube defects (raised concentration of α-fetoprotein in cell-free fluid). In the prediction of X-linked recessive disorders, when there is a 50 per cent chance of male offspring being affected, fetal sex can be determined by chromosome analysis. Individual metabolic disorders inherited as autosomal recessives are rare but some can be diagnosed prenatally by enzyme analysis of fetal cells cultured from amniotic fluid (Table 56). A helpful list of European laboratories (including those in the UK) with special experience in the biochemical diagnosis of certain inborn errors of metabolism has been compiled (Linsten *et al.* (eds) 1976).

There are many ethical implications of genetic counselling and Illingworth (1974) has drawn attention to some of them: '. . . judgement should be shown when digging deeply into the family graveyard'. The limitations of prenatal diagnosis should be explained to patients lest the procedure is misinterpreted by them as a passport for the birth of a 'perfect' baby.

The Mother and her Baby in the Maternity Hospital

Realization of pregnancy, acceptance of the fetus as a person, preparation for birth and care-giving after birth are stages in maternal adjustment that are an integral part of human reproduction. Maternal behaviour during these different stages is influenced by many environmental factors. Cultural and socioeconomic changes and modifications in obstetric policy have occurred in the last 30 years. Perhaps the most dramatic aspect of change concerns the present policy of hospital confinement (Figure 102). This has undoubtedly made childbirth safer for the mother, but at what cost? Hospital confinement has led to a change in the style of maternal care-giving from the very moment of birth and throughout the first days of life. This fact is very well known to mothers who have delivered their babies in home and hospital, but may not be apparent to our new generation of mothers. They may assume that the pattern of maternal care-giving that has evolved in the NHS maternity hospital under the supervision of the medical and nursing profession is the one most desirable for mother and baby. Fortunately the profession has recently become conscious of its responsibilities in this area. Examples of blatant thoughtlessness such as the prevention of family visiting to the maternity unit, and prolonged isolation of babies in the lying-in ward nursery are rare. However, one worrying feature of maternity-unit practice is the regimentation surrounding infant feeding schedules. The establishment and successful continuation of breast feeding is heavily influenced by the mother and baby's feeding experiences during the first week. The requirements for successful breast feeding, namely privacy, freedom which allows the mother to suckle her baby immediately her instincts compel her, together with informed guidance from a single advisor are rarely achieved in a hospital setting. The appropriate reorganization of existing rigid schedules, enabling mothers who wish to breast feed to do so under optimal conditions, is a more worthwhile approach than the coercion of unwilling mothers into breast feeding.

A subtle influence of hospital confinement on maternal care-giving is the occurrence of an inexorable train of undesirable events that may be traced back to the mother or baby being exposed to certain treatments. A case history serves as an example:

Baby A.P. Susan was a 24-year-old primigravida who in early pregnancy expressed a keen desire to breast feed her baby. Following an uncomplicated pregnancy the membranes ruptured spontaneously at term, several hours before her visit to the antenatal clinic. Examination in the clinic showed that she was draining clear liquor, the fetal head was presenting and the cervix was 'ripe'. She was admitted for induction of labour with oxytocin. Following a 12-hour labour during which she was given a combination of pethidine (150 mg) and Phenergan (25 mg) on three occasions, she gave birth to Anthony, birthweight 3.7 kg. He was rather slow to establish regular respirations and oxygen was given via a face mask. At three minutes nalorphine (0.2 mg) was given via the umbilical vein and normal respiration rapidly ensued. Susan attempted breast feeding, but Anthony would fall asleep after sucking for two or three minutes. Complementary feeds were introduced but he remained a 'slow feeder'. On the third day Anthony was examined by the paediatric resident when Susan happened to be taking a bath. The only clinical feature observed was a mild to moderate degree of jaundice. The doctor arranged for the baby to be given phototherapy forthwith. When Susan went to collect Anthony from the nursery for the 10.00 a.m. feed she was surprised to find him stripped down to his napkin, with his eyes bandaged, lying in his cot under a large piece of apparatus that was emitting a bright light. The doctor returned and consulted with Susan. He suggested that she discontinue her attempts at breast feeding because '. . . . some mothers excrete a chemical in their milk which

Table 56. Examples of disorders that may be diagnosed by biochemical analysis of fetal cells.

X-linked disorders

    Glucose-6-phosphate deficiency
    Hunter's syndrome
    Lesch–Nyhan syndrome
    Fabry's disease

Autosomal recessive disorders

    Glycogen storage disease
    Galactosaemia
    Homocystinuria
    Tach–Sachs disease
    Niemann–Pick disease
    Argininosuccinic aciduria
    Citrullinaemia

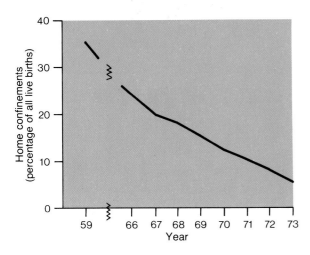

Figure 102. *Incidence of home confinements in Great Britain, 1959 to 1973.*

causes jaundice'. He stressed that jaundiced babies receiving phototherapy require a lot of fluid and because Anthony was still a little slow at feeds he would need to be fed by a nasogastric tube for a while. Following an anxious seven days in hospital Susan went home with her healthy non-jaundiced baby who was being bottle fed.

Comment. The purpose is not to criticize any particular decision but to suggest that each decision that was taken to resolve a particular problem created a further problem (Figure 103). The exposure of a mother and her baby to certain 'treatments' may have complex and subtle consequences that are not always appreciated. There was also a serious failure of communication between the professions and Susan leading to the shock of finding her baby exposed to a form of treatment she had never seen before.

The Special Care Baby Unit

Nearly 90 per cent of babies who are less than 2.5 kg at birth spend some time in a Special Care Baby Unit (SCBU) with an average length of stay of 19 days (DHSS 1971). Babies of very low birthweight (<1.5 kg), particularly those requiring intensive care, may spend the first three months of their lives in hospital.

Studies made in a variety of animals including newly born lambs and goats have shown that a short period of maternal deprivation in the first few hours of life profoundly disturbs subsequent mothering behaviour (Hersher *et al.* 1963; Moore 1968). It is now clear that maternal deprivation of the kind liable to occur when babies are cared for in an SCBU adversely influences maternal attitudes to care-giving and later development in infancy. The relatively high incidence of the 'failure to thrive' syndrome and child abuse in prematurely born babies who have been cared for in SCBUs is particularly disturbing (Klaus and Kennell 1970; Shaheen *et al.* 1968).

Figure 103. *Sequence of events likely to occur as a result of exposure to certain forms of treatment in a maternity hospital.*

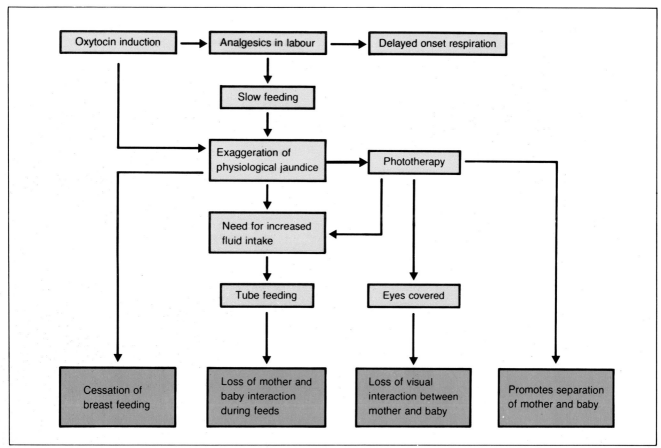

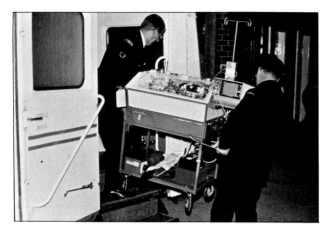

Figure 104. *Portable incubator containing patient monitoring device and resuscitation equipment being loaded into the ambulance.*

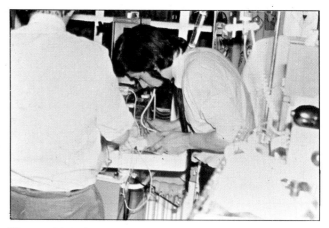

Figure 105. *At the referring hospital, stabilization of the baby's condition often involving the use of resuscitative procedures is mandatory before transfer to the neonatal intensive care unit.*

Figure 106. *Intensive care facilities including patient monitoring apparatus are available during the journey from the referring hospital to the neonatal intensive care unit.*

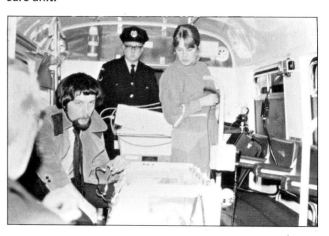

The observation of a 23 per cent incidence of mothering disorders including child abuse in mothers who visited the SCBU infrequently compared with an incidence of 1.8 per cent in mothers who were frequent visitors (Fanaroff *et al.* 1972) has special relevance. It should be possible to identify those mothers at risk of developing serious care-giving disorders by awareness of the maternal visiting pattern.

Neonatal care that only focuses on the baby is incomplete, and one must consider methods of encouraging maternal–baby interaction, allaying parental anxiety and fostering good relationships between the SCBU staff and patients. The following is a guide issued by the author to the staff on the SCBU at St Mary's Hospital, Manchester:

1. If a baby has to be admitted to the SCBU, explain to the parents in simple terms the reason for admission.

2. Explain precisely where the SCBU is situated within the maternity hospital complex. A disturbing situation for mothers is not knowing where their child is geographically, a reaction that usually persists throughout the mother's lifetime.

3. There are rarely any contraindications to parental visiting, however ill their baby is.

4. Forewarn the parents if the baby is being exposed to a form of treatment involving apparatus, e.g. incubator care, mechanical ventilation, phototherapy, etc.

5. Explain simply the function of each piece of apparatus.

6. Do not allow parents to stand away from the incubator craning to catch a glimpse of their baby. Encourage them to wash their hands and fondle their baby. The fact that their baby is attached to a mechanical ventilator is no contraindication.

7. If there are rooming-in facilities available they should be offered to parents. Remember that rooming-in by itself does not automatically bring about parental–baby interaction and there are serious emotional hazards when parents isolate themselves in their room on the SCBU.

8. Never refer to a baby as 'it', even in the parents' absence, instead use the baby's Christian name. If the parents have other children, express an interest in them and their welfare during this stressful period.

9. If asked about the baby's long-term prospects, err on the side of optimism. Never give a bad prognosis merely for fear of an unfavourable reception from the parents should the baby unexpectedly develop abnormally.

10. At some time a mother will be involved in feeding her baby on the SCBU. Before her baby is well enough to suck it is helpful if the mother can provide expressed breast milk. When her baby is able to suck, whether from a bottle or breast, feed time is of special relevance in providing the circumstances for optimal mother–baby interaction. Never cut short this period of contact merely because her baby has taken the 'required quantity' of milk. This practice would be like the waiter putting the chairs on the table just when you are enjoying the coffee after a late meal.

Regionalization of Intensive Care and the Neonatal Flying Squad

Certain very ill neonates require intensive care involving particular skills and technology that are rarely available in SCBUs. Mechanical ventilation and total parenteral nutrition are examples of intensive care techniques. The cost of providing a neonatal intensive care service is very high and it would be undesirable economically for every SCBU to be equipped and staffed for this purpose. Each unit serving a maternity hospital that catered for 2,000 births per year might only gain the experience of providing intensive care for about 10 patients each year.

During the present decade certain countries have explored the concept of the regionalisation of perinatal care and considerable progress has been made in the USA and Canada. Regional perinatal programmes involve the recognition of basic concepts that other developed countries such as the UK have been slow to accept. For example, the continuum of fetal and postnatal life is such that the concentration of neonatal intensive care resources must be closely associated with the evolution of a special type of maternity unit that caters for the referral from other maternity hospitals of women with certain antenatal problems. A three-tier system of maternal and perinatal facilities is evolving in the USA: level I units are isolated units that provide care for uncomplicated pregnancies and exist because of geographical necessity; level II units provide care for uncomplicated pregnancies and for most pregnancy complications; level III units are referral centres that provide maternal and perinatal intensive care.

In the UK, the Report of the Committee on Child Health Services (1976) stressed that at least one neonatal intensive care unit, staffed and equipped according to previous recommendations (DHSS 1971), should serve each health region (there are 14 health regions in England). The maternity unit with intensive care facilities should be one specialising in 'high risk' pregnancies where serious neonatal problems can to some extent be anticipated. Certain obstacles stand in the way of regionalisation of perinatal care in the UK, not the least being that the DHSS does not recognise perinatology or neonatology as a specialty and there are therefore no formal medical training programmes in these fields. Generally, the idea of a woman with pregnancy complications being referred from one maternity hospital to another which might have better perinatal facilities is almost taboo. Neonates in the majority of maternity hospitals in the UK are cared for by consultant paediatricians who have heavy responsibilities for general paediatric wards in hospitals that are sometimes widely separated from the maternity hospital, and rarely is there a resident paediatrician permanently available *on the premises* of the maternity hospital. Seriously ill neonates born outside maternity hospitals with neonatal intensive care facilities, particularly premature babies with respiratory problems, need the services of a flying squad to transport them safely to the neonatal intensive care unit. Indeed a safe flying squad arrangement is the core

of a neonatal intensive care service. Opposition to the regionalisation of intensive care often springs from uncertainty about the safety of transportation. Past experience has shown that *under suboptimal conditions* ill premature babies are poor travellers.

The arrangements for safe transportation at the author's hospital involve a trained doctor and nurse travelling in an ambulance to the referring hospital, taking with them a specially equipped portable incubator with a built-in mechanical ventilator (Vickers Ltd) and other monitoring devices (Figure 104). Intensive care is commenced on arrival at the referring hospital with attempts to control and stabilize the baby's condition (Figure 105), and is continued during the return journey to the intensive care unit (Figure 106).

Data from Canada clearly illustrate how the regionalisation of perinatal intensive care can markedly reduce perinatal mortality (Usher 1977). In the UK, if a neonatal flying squad and intensive care service were properly instituted in each health region, one could expect a reduction in the neonatal mortality rate in each region of about two per 1,000. This may not seem impressive but it does represent a 20 per cent reduction. It means that in absolute terms 50 to 140 lives would be saved per year in each region according to its live birth rate and that some 1,300 lives would be saved in England and Wales each year (based on birth figures for 1974). Perhaps of greater importance to society is the reasonable supposition that for every life saved a further two babies who might otherwise survive handicapped would survive intact. A sense of perspective is helpful to understand the significance of these figures even if it means making invidious comparisons. In numerical terms the results achieved by a successful neonatal intensive care service would be equivalent to at least 50 per cent of babies with myelomeningoceles surviving with every chance of developmental normality.

References

Boué, J., Boué, A. & Lazar, P., Ageing Gametes, in *International Symposium*, Seattle, p.330, Karger, Basel, 1975.

DHSS, *Report of the Expert Group on Special Care for Babies*, HMSO, London, 1971.

Fanaroff, A. A., Kennell, J. H. & Klaus, M., *Pediatrics,* 1972, **49**, 287.

Grouchy, J. de, *Aspects of Genetics in Paediatrics*, Unigate Paediatric Workshops No. 3 (Ed. Barltrop, D.), p.7, Fellowship of Postgraduate Medicine, London, 1976.

Hersher, L., Richmond, J. & Moore, A., *Behaviour*, 1963, **20**, 311.

Illingworth, R. S., in *Modern Trends in Paediatrics*, No. 4, p. 351 (Ed. Apley, J.), Butterworths, London, 1974.

Klaus, M. & Kennell, J., *Pediat. Clin. N. Amer.*, 1970, **17**, 1015.

Linsten, J., Zetterström, R. & Ferguson-Smith, M., *Acta Paediat. Scand.*, 1976, Suppl. **259**, 61.

Moore, A., in *Early Experience and Behaviour* (Ed. Newton, G. & Levine, S.), p. 481, Charles C. Thomas, Springfield, Illinois, 1968.

Report of the Committee on Child Health Services, *Fit for the Future*, HMSO, London, 1976.

Shaheen, E., Alexander, D., Truskowsky, M. & Barbero, G., *Clin. Pediat.*, 1968, **7**, 255.

Usher, R., Regionalization of perinatal care, in *Seminars in Perinatology*, 1977, **1**, 309.

Further Reading

Klaus, M. H. and Kennell, J. H., *Maternal–Infant Bonding,*
C. V. Mosby, St Louis, 1976.

Milunzky, A., Antenatal diagnosis of genetic disorders, in
Diseases of the Newborn (Ed.) Schaffer, A. J. and Avery, M. E.,
W. B. Saunders, London, Philadelphia, 1977.

Stewart, A. L., Turcan, D. M., Rawlings, G. and Reynolds,
E. G. R., *Arch. Dis. Childh.*, 1977, **52,** 97.

Index